Overcoming Metabolic Syndrome

SCOTT ISAACS, M.D.

FRED VAGNINI, M.D.

Addicus Books, Inc.
Omaha, Nebraska

An Addicus Nonfiction Book

ISBN# 1-886039-73-9

Cover design by Peri Poloni-Gabriel
Illustration by Jack Kusler
Typography by Linda Dageforde

This book is not intended to serve as a substitute for a physician. Nor is it the authors' intent to give medical advice contrary to that of an attending physician.

Library of Congress Cataloging-in-Publication Data

Isaacs, Scott, 1967-
Overcoming metabolic syndrome / Scott Isaacs, Fred Vagnini.
p. cm.
"An Addicus nonfiction book."
Includes index.
ISBN 1-886039-73-9 (alk. paper)
1. Metabolic syndrome—Popular works. I. Vagnini, Frederic J. II. Title.

RC662.4.I73 2006
616.3'9—dc22
2005024962

Addicus Books, Inc.
P.O. Box 45327
Omaha, Nebraska 68145
www.AddicusBooks.com

Printed in the United States of America
10 9 8 7 6 5 4 3 2 1

Contents

Acknowledgments

I would like to thank all my patients, past and present, for the knowledge they have given me about the multiple faces of metabolic syndrome, and for the privilege of being involved in their care. I would also like to thank my office staff: Kelli O'Neil, M.S., R.D., L.D.; Janet Baldwin, R.N.; Jennifer Truda, Melva Baker, R.N., M.S., F.N.P.B.C.; Andrea Floyd; Deborah English; and Fran Ritter, R.N.

Also, an extra special thanks to my office manager, Jennifer Steady, without whose hard work and support this book would not be possible. I would also like to thank all the nurses in the diabetes units at Northside Hospital and St. Joseph's Hospital for taking care of all my patients. I am also thankful to everyone at Addicus Books, especially Rod Colvin, for his faith in me and willingness to publish a book on this topic. I thank Todd Leopold for his editorial help.

I'd like to thank my family, Howard Isaacs, Sheryle Isaacs, Lori Johns, and Chase Johns. Finally, I'd like to thank my beautiful wife, Fiona Farrelly, who has helped me with every aspect of this book, including giving me the love and support to see this project through to completion.

Scott Isaacs, M.D.

My sincere thanks to Rod Colvin of Addicus Books for allowing me to participate in this extremely important project. I have been working on insulin resistance over the last fifteen years and was pleased to have this opportunity to work on something that has now become an American epidemic. It also represents an opportunity for health care practitioners and patients alike to prevent the complications of cardiovascular disease, diabetes, and obesity. Special thanks to my coauthor, Scott Isaacs, and for the editorial help of Todd Leopold.

I would also like to thank all of my employees at the Heart, Diabetes, and Weight Loss Centers of New York for their commitment to excellence and their help in caring for the thousands of patients that I have seen over the last twenty-five years. Special thanks also to my wonderful daughters, Grace and Clare Vagnini, for their love and understanding in my work. Special thanks also go to the founders of the American Academy of Anti-Aging Medicine, Dr. Ronald Klatz and Dr. Robert Goldman, for allowing me to present my work at the American Academy of Aging meetings. They have had the foresight to realize that insulin resistance and metabolic syndrome represent a target area to prevent the degenerative aging process.

I would also like to thank David Bunnell, CEO and founder of LongLifeClub.com, for his interest in anti-aging medicine and for allowing me to present my work over the last few years.

Fred Vagnini, M.D.

Introduction

Metabolic syndrome could be considered the new "silent epidemic," one of those conditions that affects many people but one that we don't hear too much about. As you will learn in this book, metabolic syndrome, a collection of interrelated disorders, affects millions of Americans. It is a primary contributor to our nation's growing battle with heart disease, diabetes, and other serious diseases. Chances are you will be hearing more and more about metabolic syndrome in the media. Fortunately, as the syndrome affects more people, it is gaining increasing attention.

There is good news: you can overcome this syndrome. There's no single cure, but there are ways to reverse it. Our hope is that this book will help you understand metabolic syndrome and develop strategies for escaping its grasp. Knowledge, followed by action, is the key to living a healthier, more active life.

Part 1

Understanding Metabolic Syndrome

He who has health has hope,
and he who has hope has everything.
—Arabian Proverb

1

Metabolic Syndrome: An Overview

Perhaps you have heard of metabolic syndrome. Or maybe you're like millions of others who have never heard of it. Certainly, it has not been a condition that grabs headlines like diseases such as cancer or coronary heart disease. But still, it's a serious health condition. Without lifestyle changes and treatment, it increases your risk of an early death from a heart attack or a stroke.

How prevalent is metabolic syndrome? It is estimated that 55 million Americans have metabolic syndrome. That's 27 percent of the population. Fortunately, metabolic syndrome is receiving more and more recognition as a serious medical condition, and more health professionals are diagnosing it.

What Is Metabolic Syndrome?

First, the term *metabolism* refers to the chemical and physical changes that take place within the body and enable its continued growth and functioning. A syndrome is a cluster of symptoms that characterize a specific disease or condition. However, metabolic syndrome is not actually a disease in the usual sense of the word; rather, it is a cluster of disorders. So, it would be technically inaccurate to refer to metabolic syndrome as having symptoms. Accordingly, to define it, we must look at the disorders or components that make up the syndrome.

You may have heard metabolic syndrome also being referred to by other names. It was called *syndrome X* in the years before the medical community fully understood the condition and the complex relationship between the disorders. It has also been referred to as *insulin resistance syndrome,* because insulin resistance is a core factor in the development of the condition.

Criteria for Metabolic Syndrome

There is some disagreement in the medical community over what constitutes metabolic syndrome; however, medical experts have established criteria of disorders that one must meet to be diagnosed with metabolic syndrome. Anyone with three or more of the abnormalities listed in the criteria is considered to have the syndrome.

- *High fasting blood glucose.* This means blood sugar, or glucose, levels are high when tested after fasting but are not high enough to be classified as diabetes. High glucose levels are often a sign of insulin resistance, the body's inability to use insulin efficiently.
- *Abdominal obesity.* Having fat around the belly, or "central obesity," is a key risk factor.
- *Low HDL cholesterol.* High-density lipoprotein cholesterol, or HDL, is commonly known as the "good" cholesterol.

- *High triglycerides.* Triglycerides are a form of fat the body uses for energy. The medical term for high triglycerides is *hypertriglyceridemia.*
- *High blood pressure.* High blood pressure occurs when the force of blood flowing through the artery walls is too high. High blood pressure is also referred to as *hypertension.*

This definition, or these criteria, for metabolic syndrome is the most commonly accepted one in medical circles. It was developed by the National Cholesterol Education Program of the National Heart, Lung, and Blood Institute.

Other Factors in Metabolic Syndrome

Although having high levels of low-density lipoprotein cholesterol, more commonly called LDL—the "bad" cholesterol—is not among the key criteria for metabolic syndrome, medical experts say it must be taken into consideration. Why? Because it is an "aggravating" factor, in that it increases the risk for heart attack and stroke.

Other conditions may also play a role in the development of the syndrome. One such condition is inflammation in the lining of artery walls, which may be caused by being

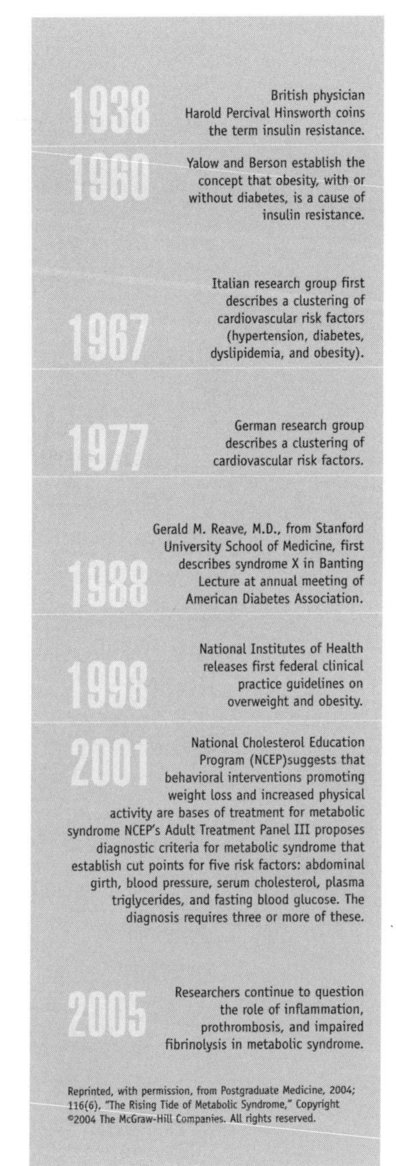

overweight, having high cholesterol, or having a chronic low-level infection. It appears such inflammation can damage the lining of artery walls and raise a person's risk for heart disease and stroke.

Another factor that may play a role in metabolic syndrome is an increased tendency to form blood clots, a process referred to as *procoagulation.* Yet another factor is an impairment in the body's ability to keep naturally occurring blood clots from growing and causing blockages. The medical term for this is *impaired fibrinolysis.*

Disorders of Metabolic Syndrome Are Interrelated

Part of what makes metabolic syndrome complex is the way in which each of the disorders influences, or "aggravates," the others. For example, insulin resistance can cause abnormal blood fats (cholesterol), high blood pressure, and high blood sugar. Similarly, high blood sugar can cause abnormal cholesterol levels. Another component of the syndrome, excessive belly fat, can result in an increase in blood sugar levels and blood pressure. In the end, the combined effect of these disorders further increases the risk of complications, which can be life threatening.

Who Gets Metabolic Syndrome?

We know that as many as 27 percent of American adults fit the criteria for the syndrome. And some experts believe that 40 percent of adults in their sixties and seventies are affected by the condition; other experts believe that as many as half the population over age sixty have metabolic syndrome.

Perhaps not surprisingly, the incidence of metabolic syndrome is increasing among young people as more and more of the nation's youth become overweight. It's estimated that 6 percent of teens, ages twelve to nineteen, meet the criteria for the syndrome.

Also, the incidence of metabolic syndrome is higher in certain ethnic groups. In the United States, Mexican Americans have a higher incidence of metabolic syndrome. Other groups that have a higher incidence are Latinos, African Americans, Native Americans, Asian Americans, and Pacific Islanders.

What Causes Metabolic Syndrome?

Just as metabolic syndrome is not one specific disease, there is not one specific cause of it. However, many medical experts consider insulin resistance to be the central defect leading to the syndrome. (You'll gain a better understanding of insulin resistance in the next chapter.) At the same time, obesity and physical inactivity play a role in the development of metabolic syndrome. Other metabolic malfunctions are likely caused by a person's genetic makeup. Aging is also a factor—as one ages, one's risk for developing the condition increases.

Can You Overcome Metabolic Syndrome?

Yes, you can. Although the complications from metabolic syndrome can be very serious, even life threatening, being diagnosed with the condition is not a death sentence. The syndrome can be reversed. Two of the most important things you can do are lose weight and increase physical activity. Additionally, medications are available to treat some of the disorders. We will be covering these topics throughout the book.

2

The Disorders of Metabolic Syndrome: A Closer Look

Every year, metabolic syndrome becomes more of a public health threat. Why? Because it increases the chances of death from cardiovascular disease. Interestingly, deaths from cardiovascular disease have declined over the past fifty years. This is due largely to improved emergency care in our nation's hospitals, as well as to improved clinical care and public health efforts to reduce the risk of disease. However, given the increasing trend toward obesity and metabolic syndrome in the past two decades, the progress in lowering the death rate due to cardiovascular disease could be reversed.

To avoid becoming one of the unfortunate statistics, you should be aware of two key points. The first is understanding the disorders that make up metabolic syndrome. The second is knowing which syndromes affect you and how you can overcome them.

In this chapter, we'll take a closer look at criteria for metabolic syndrome:

- High fasting blood glucose levels

- Abdominal obesity
- Low HDL cholesterol
- High triglycerides
- High blood pressure

Disorder: High Fasting Blood Glucose Levels

It's estimated that 41 million Americans between the ages of 40 and 74 have abnormal blood glucose (sugar) levels. When you have high levels of sugar in your blood, it means your body is not metabolizing sugars adequately. Four outcomes are possible when your blood sugar levels are tested:

- *Normal level*: Your blood sugar level is in the normal range, meaning your body's insulin is keeping your sugar level under control.
- *Impaired fasting glucose*: blood sugar values during fasting are above normal but not high enough to be classified as diabetes.
- *Impaired glucose tolerance*: Blood sugar values are above normal after drinking a sugar solution during a glucose tolerance test but do not meet the criteria for a diagnosis of diabetes.
- *Type 2 diabetes*: Blood sugar values meet the criteria for diabetes.

From High Blood Sugar to Insulin Resistance

If your doctor tells you that you have high blood sugar, chances are you have been gradually becoming insulin resistant for some time. In fact, the earliest stages of insulin resistance occur many years before a person develops blood sugar problems. To fully understand metabolic syndrome, it is important to understand insulin resistance. In the simplest terms, insulin resistance is a condition in which the body is not able to properly use insulin to move glucose from the blood into cells and convert it to energy.

How Does Insulin Resistance Develop?

Here's how the process works. When you eat, glucose is released into the bloodstream, making your blood sugar level rise. The job of the hormone insulin—which is produced by beta cells in the pancreas—is to move the sugar from the blood into the body's cells to be used for energy. Once that is done, your blood sugar level returns to normal. But when you have insulin resistance, the cells in your body are impaired and are less efficient at using insulin. It is as if your body doesn't recognize the insulin or know how to use it—your body resists the insulin.

When insulin is not efficient at moving glucose into cells for energy, the body tries to compensate by stimulating the pancreas to produce yet more insulin. Eventually, as the body tries to produce more and more insulin to bring blood sugar under control, the beta cells in the pancreas wear out.

This series of actions leads to weight gain. The higher insulin levels stimulate appetite centers in the brain and increase hunger. Furthermore, insulin is a fat storage hormone, so higher insulin levels mean that more of the calories consumed are converted to fat instead of burned as energy. This sets up a vicious cycle of weight gain, increased insulin resistance, higher insulin levels, increased appetite, and more fat storage. The end result is elevated blood sugars, which can lead to type 2 diabetes.

If you have impaired fasting glucose or impaired glucose tolerance, you are said to have "prediabetes." It is important to know this and take actions to reverse it, because prediabetes means your pancreas is already starting to show signs of strain. Even when blood sugar is minimally elevated, the condition can begin causing damage to the heart and circulatory system. Symptoms of elevated blood sugar may be nonexistent at first. If the condition is not diagnosed promptly, you will eventually experience symptoms of diabetes—excessive thirst, excessive hunger, frequent urination, and blurred vision.

The Pancreas

The pancreas, an organ about the size of a hand, is located behind the lower part of the stomach. Two types of cells are found throughout the pancreas: alpha cells, which make *glucagon*, a hormone that raises the level of glucose (sugar) in the blood, and *beta cells*, which make insulin.

Causes of Insulin Resistance

Researchers trying to find the causes of insulin resistance have found a variety of problems in the most basic workings of cells. And even though there is much that is still unknown about insulin resistance, the medical community has identified several causes.

- *Obesity.* This is the most common cause of insulin resistance. Most individuals become insulin resistant when they are 35 to 40 percent above their ideal body weight. Being overweight overloads tissues with excess fatty acids in the blood and promotes insulin resistance.

- *Genetics.* Your family history is a key factor. In fact, genetics determine at what weight you *will* develop insulin resistance, rather than *whether* you will develop it.
- *Physical inactivity.* A sedentary lifestyle promotes a multitude of metabolic changes that contribute to metabolic syndrome.
- *Stress.* When the body is stressed, the adrenal glands release a hormone called *cortisol.* An excess of this hormone is thought to play a part in the development of insulin resistance. Individuals with too much cortisol often develop upper-body fat, which can influence the development of metabolic syndrome. Cortisol also can stimulate appetite and cause weight gain.
- *Cigarette smoking.* This is known to increase insulin resistance.
- *Infection or illness.* These may increase or decrease production of hormones key to insulin production and processing.
- *Pregnancy.* The fluctuation of hormones in pregnancy may influence insulin production and blood sugar levels.

Complications of Insulin Resistance

The complications that can arise out of insulin resistance are essentially the same as those that can result from metabolic syndrome. Any of the complications can be quite serious; however, the combined effect of the disorders intensifies the risk of heart attack or stroke.

Cardiovascular Disease

This is the most serious and most feared complication of metabolic syndrome. It is the number one cause of death in the United States. Cardiovascular disease includes heart attacks and strokes, but any organ can be affected. Cardiovascular disease is a general term that refers to diseases of the heart and blood vessels caused by *atherosclerosis*. Also referred to as "hardening of the arteries," atherosclerosis is a process by which deposits of cholesterol, called plaques, build up in the arteries. There are several major forms of cardiovascular disease:

- Coronary artery disease, which leads to heart attacks
- Carotid artery disease, which leads to strokes
- Peripheral arterial disease, which is atherosclerosis in the blood vessels of the legs, which can lead to an amputation
- Renal vascular disease, which can lead to kidney failure

Type 2 Diabetes

This is the end stage of insulin resistance, and it occurs when insulin-producing cells in the pancreas are worn out—they finally stop functioning. Many people have insulin resistance for ten years or longer before they know it, and may have diabetes for five years or longer before they are finally diagnosed. Early on, when the body is not able to use insulin adequately (insulin resistance), the pancreas secretes enough additional insulin to overcome the resistance; however, over time the pancreas can become "exhausted," and supply cannot keep up with demand. This is when blood sugar levels rise.

Diabetes can bring about serious complications, including cardiovascular disease. Heart attacks and strokes occur four times as frequently in people with diabetes as in people without diabetes. Diabetes is also the most common cause of kidney failure and blindness in adults. Other potential complications: nerve damage, which may lead to pain and numbness in the hands and feet, and damage to blood vessels, which may result in amputation of limbs. Nerve damage also may cause digestive problems and sexual dysfunction.

Left Ventricular Hypertrophy

This condition is marked by an abnormal thickening of the part of the heart responsible for pumping blood throughout the body. When the heart muscle is overworked, it enlarges, much as your biceps would from lifting weights, but an enlarged, more muscular heart muscle is not healthy. The heart muscle grows in an effort to help the heart do its work; however, over time the thickened muscle actually becomes stiff, loses flexibility, and fails to pump adequate volumes of blood. Left ventricular hypertrophy is best diagnosed with an electrocardiogram (EKG) or an echocardiogram, an ultrasound test of the heart in action. This condition is often treated by controlling high blood pressure.

Obstructive Sleep Apnea

This disorder involves blockage of the airway and is often related to obesity; in the simplest of terms, when a person lies flat, fat tissue can obstruct the airway. The disorder is more likely to occur in men with a neck circumference greater than seventeen inches and in women with a neck circumference greater than sixteen inches.

To an observer, an individual with sleep apnea snores loudly and has episodes in which breathing stops, followed by gasps or snorts when the person is awakened by the apnea. These sleep disruptions result in chronic fatigue. Sleep apnea is linked to heart rhythm disturbances, heart attack and stroke, and sudden death. Sleep apnea is best diagnosed in a sleep laboratory, where electrodes monitor sleeping habits. In-home evaluations are also available but are not always accurate.

Sleep apnea can be treated with a CPAP machine, an instrument that acts as a "breathing mask" and provides a smooth, continuous flow of oxygen to the sleeper. In extreme cases, surgery to widen the airway may be required.

Fatty Liver Disease

This is also known as *nonalcoholic steatohepatosis (NASH) or nonalcoholic fatty liver disease (NAFLD).* This disease of the liver is similar to that caused by excessive use of alcohol; however, alcohol is not involved. The condition is marked by fat in the liver, along with inflammation and liver damage. Many people are unaware they have this condition; however, if their disease progresses, it can cause permanent scarring, known as *cirrhosis of the liver.* Blood tests that show elevated liver enzymes often indicate this liver problem. Other diagnostic tests include ultrasound and CT scan. In rare cases, a liver biopsy is required; this involves using a needle to remove a tiny piece of liver tissue, which a pathologist examines. Treatment involves weight loss, physical activity, and proper nutrition.

Acanthosis Nigricans

This is a very common skin condition that appears as a black or dark discoloration with a velvety appearance. It looks like dirt, but it won't wash off. Acanthosis nigricans commonly occurs on the neck, under the arms, or in the groin. This condition is a direct result of insulin resistance and obesity. It is frequently a sign of prediabetes or diabetes.

Pregnancy Problems

Metabolic syndrome is associated with an increased risk for gestational diabetes and high blood pressure in pregnancy, known as preeclampsia.

Polycystic Ovary Syndrome

A hormonal disorder (PCOS) is believed to affect some 10 million women in the United States. Insulin resistance stimulates the ovaries and adrenal glands to produce excess male hormones, resulting in irregular menstrual cycles, fertility problems, acne, and facial hair growth. If not managed, PCOS can lead to diabetes, cardiovascular disease, and *endometrial hyperplasia*, a condition caused by the buildup of old cells in the *endometrium*, the lining of the uterus. Endometrial hyperplasia may lead to uterine cancer. PCOS is diagnosed by hormonal blood testing and ultrasound examination of the ovaries.

Male Hormone Problems

Men with metabolic syndrome are at high risk for low testosterone, known as *hypogonadism*, which is associated with muscle loss, fatigue, depression, and sexual dysfunction. Male hypogonadism is diagnosed with blood tests for levels of the hormone testosterone.

Gout

Gout is a painful disorder characterized by uric acid deposits in the joints, most commonly the big toe. Metabolic syndrome causes increased levels of uric acid and can lead to gout. Increased uric acid levels have also been associated with an increased risk of cardiovascular disease. Gout is best diagnosed by drawing a small amount of fluid from an inflamed joint.

Kidney Disease

Metabolic syndrome increases the risk for protein leakage from the kidney and chronic renal failure. Early kidney disease can be diagnosed with a urine test that measures microscopic amounts of protein in the urine, known as microalbumin. It is recommended that all patients with metabolic syndrome have urine microalbumin testing at least once or twice a year.

Gallbladder Disease

Metabolic syndrome increases the risk for gallstones and the need for gallbladder removal. Gallbladder disease can be diagnosed with an ultrasound of the gallbladder.

Psychiatric Problems

People with metabolic syndrome frequently have problems such as depression or anxiety.

Cancer

Metabolic syndrome increases the risk for a variety of cancers, including cancers of the colon, breast, uterus, and prostate.

Increased Risk of Blood Clotting

Metabolic syndrome elevates the risk of blood clots, which in turn increase the chances of having a heart attack, stroke, or blood clots in the legs, known as *deep vein thrombosis* (*DVT*).

Disorder: Abdominal Obesity

The United States is experiencing an epidemic of obesity. More than half the population is overweight, and 35 percent are considered obese. When we are obese, the extra weight puts a strain on the body's heart and organs. The heart, for example, is required to pump blood to all the additional fat tissue throughout the body. However, among all the risk factors for metabolic syndrome, abdominal obesity—excessive belly fat—is the most important.

Why is abdominal fat such an important factor? Although the exact reasons that this fat is so critical are not fully understood, medical experts believe that belly fat is very active metabolically and contains cells, called *adipocytes*, that release fatty acids and other hormones into the bloodstream; this action causes an increase in insulin resistance. In addition, the abdominal fat cells produce toxic chemicals, called *cytokines*. These chemicals disrupt the normal production of insulin and may promote chronic inflammation of tissues and the lining of blood vessels. In turn, these actions may also increase insulin resistance, which may promote high blood pressure and abnormal cholesterol levels. Regardless of the exact biological process that occurs, the research is clear: abdominal fat is an important risk factor in metabolic syndrome, and the amount of fat influences the degree of insulin resistance.

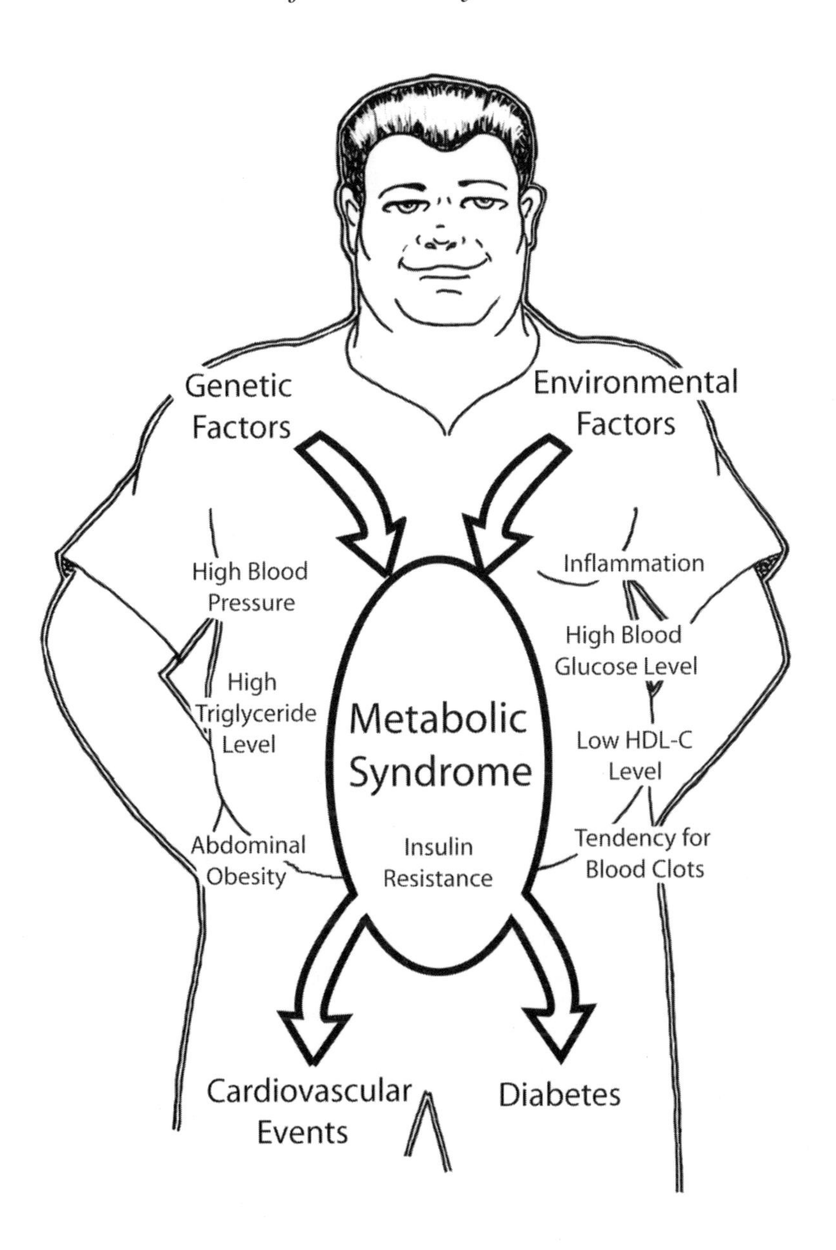
Genetic Factors
Environmental Factors
High Blood Pressure
Inflammation
High Blood Glucose Level
High Triglyceride Level
Metabolic Syndrome
Low HDL-C Level
Tendency for Blood Clots
Abdominal Obesity
Insulin Resistance
Cardiovascular Events
Diabetes

Disorder: Low HDL—the "Good" Cholesterol

People with obesity and insulin resistance often have abnormal levels of blood fats, including low high-density lipoproteins (HDL). Before discussing HDL cholesterol, let's take a broader look at blood fats.

It is normal to have fats circulating in the bloodstream. These fats are also known as *lipids* or *lipoproteins.* You're probably more familiar with the term cholesterol than with lipids or blood fats. And you're probably used to hearing about cholesterol in a negative way. However, cholesterol itself is not a bad thing. It serves a useful purpose in the body. It works in the bloodstream to help produce cellular membranes, aids in hormone production, and performs a variety of other functions.

The two primary types of cholesterol are *high-density lipoprotein* (HDL) cholesterol and *low-density lipoprotein* (LDL) cholesterol. Having abnormal levels of these cholesterols is known as *dyslipidemia.* Most people know that high LDL cholesterol is a risk factor for cardiovascular disease, but research has shown that low HDL is an even greater risk factor for developing heart and blood vessel problems.

HDL Cholesterol

HDL cholesterol is considered the "good" cholesterol. It acts as a scavenger as it travels through the bloodstream, eating away at harmful cholesterol and carrying it away from the arteries and on into the liver for excretion from the body. This action prevents the formation of clogged arteries. So, when HDL levels are too low, it is not able to do its job.

But did you know there are several forms, or subtypes, of HDL? The form known as HDL_2 is made up of larger particles and is considered the best type, because it provides the most protection from arteries being clogged. The subtype HDL_3 offers only moderate protection against clogging. So, the particle size of the HDL floating in your bloodstream is important. Your HDL values may appear normal, but if the particles are small and dense, you're not as well protected against cardiovascular disease.

Other than premature cardiovascular disease, there are no specific symptoms of low HDL cholesterol. However, insulin resistance is a major cause of lowered HDL levels. Other causal factors are cigarette smoking, physical inactivity, obesity, kidney disease, liver disease, diabetes, genetics, and some medications, including diuretics and beta-blocker medications. HDL can be boosted through increased physical activity and a healthful diet.

LDL Cholesterol

As mentioned previously, an elevated LDL cholesterol level is *not* a key criterion for metabolic syndrome; however, it has a significant influence on the development of the factors that do make up metabolic syndrome. And just as there are several forms of HDL, there is more than one form of LDL.

All forms are dangerous because they can cause plaques to form in artery walls; however, the particle size of the LDL determines the degree of danger. For example, pattern A, which is made up of larger, "fluffy" particles, is the least dangerous form. Pattern B is made up of small and dense, or concentrated, particles and is considered the most dangerous, because the particles are capable of easily entering artery walls and forming plaques.

People with metabolic syndrome tend to have higher levels of the pattern B LDL cholesterol. A third type of LDL, AB pattern, is made up of a combination of small and large particles and is considered to pose an intermediate level of risk.

Complications of Abnormal Blood Fats

Both HDL cholesterol and LDL cholesterol contribute to the potential complications brought on by abnormal blood fats.

- *Atherosclerosis.* This condition refers to fatty deposits in the walls of arteries. These deposits can harden and may block the arteries.
- *Coronary disease.* The type of heart disease caused by high cholesterol is usually caused by atherosclerosis. As the blood vessels narrow due to the cholesterol deposits, oxygen to the heart is diminished. Eventually, a cholesterol deposit can rupture, forming a blood clot in the vessel, leading to a heart attack.
- *Stroke.* Atherosclerosis in the blood vessels of the brain or neck can undergo a process similar to a heart attack, leading to a stroke.
- *Peripheral arterial disease.* Atherosclerosis in the blood vessels of the legs can lead to decreased blood flow and amputations.

Disorder: High Triglycerides

A high triglyceride level is yet another of the disorders that make up metabolic syndrome.

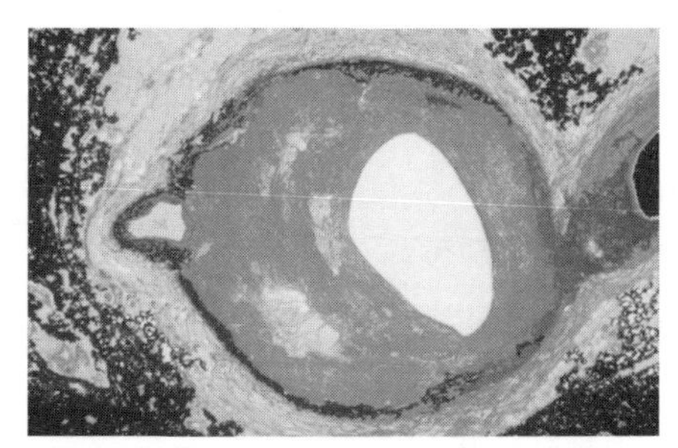

Plaque buildup obstructs the flow of the blood through the artery. The white area, in the center, represents the only portion of the artery not blocked. *Custom Medical Stock Photo.*

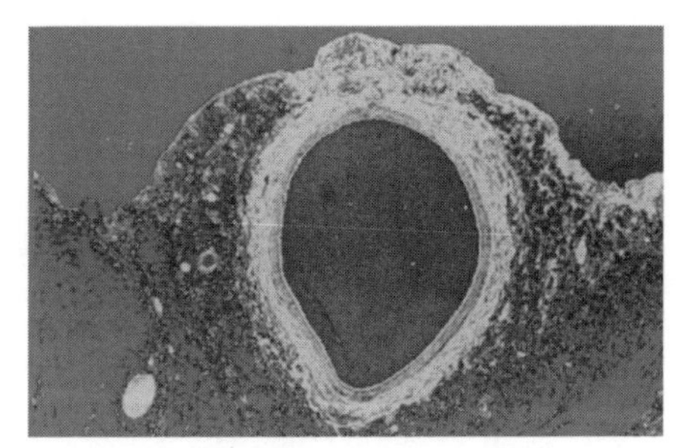

An open artery, shown above, easily transports oxygenated blood away from the heart to other parts of the body. *Custom Medical Stock Photo.*

Most of the fat in your body is composed of triglycerides. These lipids are stored in adipose tissue, or fat tissue. When the body needs energy, the adipose tissue breaks down the triglycerides and releases them into the bloodstream as fatty acids. In obese individuals, too much fatty acid is released, and tissues become overloaded with fat, contributing to insulin resistance.

Triglycerides are also the most common form of fat in your diet. The majority of fats you eat, including vegetable oil and animal products, contain triglyceride molecules. Also, carbohydrates are converted to triglycerides by the body. When you eat more than you need, the body converts the excess calories to triglycerides, which are stored as fat.

Potential Complications of High Triglycerides

- *Atherosclerosis.* When triglyceride levels in the bloodstream are too high, the fat can build up in the arteries, causing plaque, which sticks to the artery walls and clogs them, resulting in cardiovascular disease.

- *Pancreatitis.* Very high triglyceride levels (usually above 1,000 mg/dL, or milligrams per deciliter) can inflame the pancreas, resulting in this possibly life-threatening disease. Symptoms of pancreatitis include pain in the abdomen (which may occur twelve to twenty-four hours after eating a large meal or drinking alcohol heavily), nausea, vomiting, abdominal distention and tenderness, shortness of breath, fever, or rapid heartbeat. Sometimes pancreatitis can become chronic; in such case, a person may have milder symptoms and a more insidious version of the disease.
- *Eruptive xanthomas.* These are small acnelike skin lesions that may appear yellowish with a red base and are most often seen on the back, buttocks, chest, upper arms, and upper legs. Eruptive xanthomas are usually seen when triglyceride levels are above 1,000 mg/dL.
- *Eye problems.* If triglyceride levels are above 4,000 mg/dL, a condition known as *lipemia retinalis* may set in. The blood vessels in the retina may take on a pale pink, milky appearance from triglycerides in the blood, and vision problems result.
- *Neurological problems.* Triglyceride elevations have been reported to cause memory loss, dementia, and depression in some patients.

What Causes Dyslipidemia (Abnormal Blood Fat Levels)?

- *Insulin resistance.* This can result in increased fat production and is associated with high triglyceride levels and low HDL levels.
- *A diet high in fat.* Saturated fats and trans fats are especially risky.
- *Low-fat, high-carbohydrate diets.* Diets made up almost exclusively of carbohydrates can raise lipid levels.
- *Genetics.* High lipid levels tend to run in families, which is why even good nutrition, exercise, and stable weight aren't always enough to keep them low.
- *Physical inactivity.* On the other hand, exercise and physical activity improve lipid profiles, raising HDL cholesterol levels and lowering triglycerides.
- *Stress.* Elevations in cortisol, a hormone secreted by the adrenal glands when the body is under stress, promote insulin resistance and stimulate appetite and weight gain.

Disorder: High Blood Pressure

More than half of all Americans over age fifty have high blood pressure, also known as hypertension. Unfortunately, approximately half of those with high blood pressure are not being treated for it. High blood pressure cannot be cured, but it can be controlled.

Blood pressure refers to the force applied to the artery walls as the heart pumps the blood. It's measured in two forms: the pressure when the heart beats (known as the *systolic pressure*) and the pressure when the heart is at rest (*diastolic pressure*). When recording blood pressure, a health professional lists the systolic pressure, which is higher, over the diastolic pressure, which is lower. For example, normal blood pressure is 120/80 or lower.

Symptoms of high blood pressure are often nonexistent, which is why it is known as the "silent killer." Individuals can be unaware they have hypertension until they develop symptoms, such as headaches, dizziness, sleeplessness, or ringing in the ears. Those with high blood pressure also are at risk for much more serious complications, such as heart attack, stroke, or even sudden death.

Causes of High Blood Pressure

- *Aging.* The risk of high blood pressure increases with age. A form of high blood pressure common among older adults is *isolated systolic hypertension.* This refers to blood pressure in which the systolic number, or top number, is 140 or higher, but the bottom number, diastolic pressure, is normal.
- *Genetics.* Heredity is believed to play a role in up to 50 percent of cases.
- *Ethnicity.* Certain groups, such as African Americans, Latinos, and Asians, have a greater risk, as do people with heart disease, kidney disease, or liver disease. Other people may have high blood pressure because of a high-salt diet or a stressful lifestyle.
- *Atherosclerosis.* As mentioned previously, the heart works harder when trying to circulate blood through clogged arteries. This can lead to an increase in blood pressure.

- *Kidney problems.* The kidney produces hormones that regulate blood pressure. Kidney problems can result in higher levels of these hormones.
- *Insulin resistance.* Some research suggests that resistance to insulin may influence blood pressure. Insulin resistance increases the retention of sodium (salt), which may increase circulating blood fluid volume.
- *Medications.* Some drugs contribute to high blood pressure, including estrogen-containing medications, cold remedies with stimulants, some antidepressants, steroids, nonsteroidal anti-inflammatory drugs (NSAID), and asthma medications.
- *Hormonal problems.* Certain ailments—such as diabetes, thyroid problems, adrenal gland problems, and pituitary gland problems—cause high blood pressure.
- *Situational stress and tension.* An example of situational stress is "white-coat hypertension," in which a person's blood pressure is elevated in a doctor's office because he or she is anxious about the medical examination. Though once dismissed as only nervousness, white-coat hypertension is now considered a real form of hypertension because it has been found that other stressful situations may also raise blood pressure. Most experts now agree that hypertension from situational stress should be taken seriously and treated like any other type.

Potential Complications of High Blood Pressure

- *Atherosclerosis.* In persons with high blood pressure, blood vessels become narrower and less elastic, making it more difficult for blood to deliver oxygen and nutrients to organs.
- *Heart disease.* Having high blood pressure means the heart must pump harder to get the blood through the arteries. The heart enlarges, heart muscle thickens, and eventually the heart can fail. In addition, the enlarged ventricles are more prone to irregular and rapid heartbeat, or *arrhythmia.* Every twenty-point increase in your systolic (top) number or ten-point increase in your diastolic (bottom) number doubles your risk for heart attack or stroke.
- *Stroke.* High blood pressure increases a person's risk for two major types of strokes. Atherosclerosis of the blood vessels of the neck or head increases the chance that a blood clot will block the artery, thereby depriving the brain of oxygen. This is known as a *thrombotic stroke.* A *hemorrhagic stroke,* another type, also can be caused by high blood pressure; in this case, a blood vessel in the brain bursts and bleeds into the brain.
- *Peripheral arterial disease.* High blood pressure is a contributing factor to blood vessel problems in the legs.
- *Kidney failure.* High blood pressure in the kidney results in destruction of the small renal (kidney) vessels, resulting in progressive impaired renal function and possibly kidney failure. This is known as *hypertensive nephropathy.*

- *Blindness.* High blood pressure can damage the blood vessels in the eyes, a condition known as *hypertensive retinopathy.*

Understanding Promotes Action

Now that you have a better understanding of the cluster of disorders that comprise metabolic syndrome, you'll be in a better position to understand the results of the diagnostic tests your physician may perform. To overcome metabolic syndrome or any medical condition that may be taking a toll on your health, it is important that you become an informed and conscientious consumer. Only then can you take the action that will help you restore your good health.

Remember that it's okay to ask your doctor for help in understanding metabolic syndrome. There are so "silly" questions when it comes to making sure you have a clear idea of what you need to do to stave off serious, even deadly, disease.

3

Getting a Diagnosis

As you learn more about metabolic syndrome, you may find yourself wondering whether you have it. If you are already aware of your cholesterol values, blood pressure, and blood sugar levels, you may already have a sense of whether you have metabolic syndrome.

How is it diagnosed? There is no single diagnostic test that doctors can use to determine whether you have the syndrome. Essentially, you are tested for each of the disorders individually. A clinical evaluation typically involves assessing:

- Fasting blood glucose levels
- Abdominal obesity
- Lipid profiles—cholesterol and triglyceride levels
- Blood pressure

Why Is Getting a Diagnosis Important?

For most diseases, getting a diagnosis is important so that doctors can prescribe a specific treatment. However, as we have discussed, metabolic syndrome is not a single disease, and there is not one specific treatment for it. Still, it is important to know whether you have the syndrome, because of the aggravating effect each of the disorders has on the others. A lot is not understood about metabolic syndrome; however, the research is clear: having disorders that make up the syndrome significantly increases your risk of death. In fact, compared with those who don't have it, those with metabolic syndrome are 3.5 times as likely to die of a heart-related problem and 5 times as likely to develop type 2 diabetes. Research also has shown that metabolic syndrome is equal to cigarette smoking as being a risk factor for cardiovascular disease.

Who Diagnoses Metabolic Syndrome?

A number of medical professionals, from generalists to specialists, are capable of diagnosing metabolic syndrome. It is commonly diagnosed by the following physicians:

- *Primary care physician.* This could be a general practitioner, a family practitioner, a pediatrician, or an internist.
- *Endocrinologist.* This physician specializes in hormones and the glands of the endocrine system, which regulates metabolism, hunger, energy level, the menstrual cycle, and many other bodily functions.
- *Cardiologist.* This doctor specializes in the heart and vascular (blood vessels) system.

Are You at Risk for Metabolic Syndrome?

- Do you have a family history of one of the following: diabetes, obesity, high blood pressure?
- Is your blood pressure higher than 135/85?
- Are your triglycerides greater than 150?
- Is your fasting glucose above 100?
- Do you have elevated uric acid or gout?
- Are you overweight—is your body mass index 25 or more?
- Do you exercise less than ninety minutes per week? Are you inactive?
- Do you have skin tags or a darkish discoloration (acanthosis nigricans) around your neck, groin, or armpits?

For Women Only

- Do you have any history of gestational diabetes—diabetes with pregnancy?
- Have you delivered a baby nine pounds or more?
- Do you have a history of infertility, facial hair growth, adult acne, abnormal menstrual cycles, or polycystic ovary syndrome (PCOS)?
- Is your waist circumference thirty-five inches or above?
- Is your HDL cholesterol 50 or below?

For Men Only

- Is your testosterone low? Do you have any sexual dysfunction?
- Is your waist circumference forty inches or above?
- Is your HDL cholesterol 40 or below?

If you answered yes to *any* of the questions, you are at risk, and you should investigate treatments with your doctor.

Diagnosing: High Blood Sugar Levels

Doctors can determine whether your body is metabolizing sugars normally by performing a blood test that measures your blood sugar level. If your body is not using sugars normally, insulin is not working efficiently in your body. Four tests are commonly used to measure sugars, or glucose, in the blood:

- Fasting plasma glucose test
- Oral glucose tolerance test
- Hemoglobin A1c test
- Meal tolerance test

Fasting Plasma Glucose Test

The fasting plasma glucose test is the one most commonly used to check blood sugar. It is designed to determine the normal, baseline amount of glucose in your blood on an average day. The American Diabetes Association considers it the screening test of choice for diagnosing diabetes.

> *Before the test.* Fast at least six hours before taking the test. Some physicians recommend at least eight hours of fasting.
>
> *The procedure.* Blood is drawn from a vein in the arm and then tested for glucose.
>
> *Blood sugar levels.* Most medical experts have established 100 mg/dL or below as "normal."

If you have a fasting blood sugar level between 100 and 125, you are classified as having an "impaired fasting glucose" and are at high risk for type 2 diabetes, high blood pressure, high cholesterol, and other disorders related to metabolic syndrome. If your level is above 126, you are considered to have diabetes, according to the American Diabetes Association.

Another test, the plasma glucose test called the *random plasma glucose test*, can be done at any time without fasting. For this test, a normal blood sugar level is below 140. A diabetic level is more than 200.

Oral Glucose Tolerance Test

The *oral glucose tolerance test* determines how quickly and efficiently your body processes glucose. It is often used to screen pregnant women for gestational diabetes—diabetes that occurs during pregnancy—and is also frequently given to any patient who shows signs of metabolic syndrome, such as abdominal obesity or high triglycerides, or who has a family history of the syndrome's elements.

Blood Measurements—What They Mean

The standard measurement used in blood tests is listed as "mg/dL," which refers to milligrams per deciliter. A deciliter is a little less than half a cup. The body contains about six quarts, or 5.6 liters, of blood. A deciliter is 0.1 liter.

Before the test: Eat a consistent diet for three days before the test, containing between 150 and 200 grams of carbohydrates a day. Stop drinking (except water), smoking, and exercising at least eight hours before the test. Fast eight hours before the test.

Consult with your physician if you're on any medications. Among drugs that can alter results are corticosteroids, birth control pills, anticonvulsants, and some high blood pressure medications.

The Procedure. A blood sample is drawn. This creates a baseline blood sugar level with which others will be compared. You're given a beverage containing seventy-five grams of glucose. It tastes like soft drink syrup. Two hours later, your blood is drawn again and its blood sugar content compared with the baseline sample. Some doctors measure blood at hourly intervals for up to five hours, but the two-hour sample is the standard.

Fasting Blood Sugar Level Classifications

Normal:	Less than 100 mg/dL*
Impaired fasting glucose:	100 to 125 mg/dL
Diabetes:	Greater than 125 mg/dL

If blood sugar is greater than 110 mg/dL, the patient qualifies for metabolic syndrome.

*Measurements are in milligrams per liter of blood, or mg/DL.

Two-Hour Stimulated Glucose Level Classifications

- Less than 139 mg/dL: normal
- 140-199 mg/dL: impaired glucose tolerance
- Greater than 200 mg/dL: diabetes

Hemoglobin A1c Test

The *hemoglobin A1c test*—also referred to as "A1c"—calculates how blood sugar levels have acted over the past three to four months. Hemoglobin A1c is a blood protein in red blood cells that bonds with blood sugar. Because red blood cells can live from 90 to 120 days, the hemoglobin A1c stays in the blood for that length of time. Accordingly, it is effective in measuring blood sugar over a period of time. Most doctors routinely run this test every few months for people with diabetes or metabolic syndrome.

Before the test. No fasting is necessary.

The procedure. A blood sample is drawn from a vein in the arm.

Hemoglobin A1c. A normal level is less than 6 percent hemoglobin A1c; some doctors prefer an even lower level of 5.5 percent.

For now, the exact A1c levels necessary to make a diagnosis of diabetes or metabolic syndrome have not been established; however, some doctors treat patients for diabetes if the level is 5.7 or higher.

In the past, in fact, this test was recommended for only those with diabetes. More recently, however, A1c has been recognized as an excellent test for assessing long-term blood sugar levels in nondiabetic patients. Elevated A1c is also an independent risk factor for cardiovascular disease.

Meal Tolerance Test

The meal tolerance test, also known as a *postprandial blood glucose test,* determines how quickly and efficiently your body processes glucose. Many physicians do not use the test, because there are no specific food products recommended, nor is there a specific amount of sugar to be used in the meal.

Before the test. No fasting is necessary.

The procedure. The meal tolerance test is similar to the oral glucose tolerance test. First, blood is drawn and checked for glucose levels. Then, instead, drinking a sugary beverage, you eat a big meal. Two hours later, another blood sample is drawn and tested for its blood sugar level.

Glucose levels. If the blood sugar level is above 200 mg/dL, the patient is considered diabetic. If it's above 140, the patient is at risk for diabetes.

The meal tolerance test is probably the most unpredictable of the blood sugar tests, because it is full of variables that may influence the results. For this reason, it is usually part of an overall battery of tests, if it's done at all.

Testing Variables

Several factors can affect results of blood sugar tests. For example, errors may be made by the labs that perform the blood tests. Labs should be certified by the U.S. government in accordance with the Clinical Laboratory Improvement Amendments (CLIA) of 1988. For consistency, your doctor will likely use the same lab each time.

Various medications can affect blood test results; your doctor will likely ask you about medications you are taking.

Home kits are available for testing blood sugar; however, home testing kits are not as reliable as laboratory testing. When diagnosing metabolic syndrome, most physicians will look not only at blood tests but also at other criteria for metabolic syndrome.

Are Insulin Levels Tested?

Because insulin resistance is the cause of metabolic syndrome, you might think that measuring insulin levels in the blood would be helpful for diagnosing it. However, most experts do not recommend measuring insulin levels, for two reasons. First, laboratory testing methods for insulin are still unreliable and are often inaccurate. Secondly, often a person with insulin resistance actually has normal or even low insulin levels, because their pancreas has "burned out." Nevertheless, some doctors still measure insulin levels to make the diagnosis of insulin resistance. If insulin is measured, it should be after an eight-hour fast. An insulin level above 10 or 15 uU/ml is considered high.

Diagnosing: Obesity

A person's body fat status refers to the amount, type, and distribution of fat in your body. This is another feature that gives your physician an overall impression of your body's metabolic risk. To determine obesity, doctors use several "measuring sticks." These methods include body mass index (BMI), waist circumference, and body fat analysis.

Body Mass Index

The most important of the obesity measures is one's percentage of body fat as determined by the *body mass index*, or BMI. It is a ratio between one's weight and one's height. BMI is determined by the following formula:

$$\frac{\text{(weight in pounds x 703)}}{\text{(height in inches) x (height in inches)}} = \text{BMI}$$

For example, if a man weighs 190 pounds and is 5 feet 10 inches tall, his numeric formula would be:

$$\frac{190 \times 703}{\text{70 inches x 70 inches (or 4,900)}} = \text{a BMI of 27}$$

Classification of Weight by BMI

Less than 18.5	Underweight
18.5-24.9	Normal
25-29.9	Overweight
30-34.9	Class I obesity
35-39.9	Class II obesity
Greater than 40	Class III obesity
Greater than 60	Super-obesity

Using BMI does have its drawbacks. The formula doesn't consider lean body mass, so a muscular, heavy person may have a high BMI but be in terrific shape. However, for the vast majority of the population, BMI remains the best overall indicator of obesity.

Waist Circumference

Another quick and easy way to assess obesity is measuring waist circumference. Public health experts have noted there is a strong correlation between waist circumference and metabolic syndrome and other conditions—cardiovascular disease and type 2 diabetes.

To properly measure waist circumference, place a tape measure comfortably around your body, in the smallest area below the rib cage and above the navel. Men with a waist measurement greater than forty inches, and women with a waist measurement above thirty-five inches, fit the control obesity criteria for metabolic syndrome.

Some physicians also recommend measuring the circumference around the hips and noting the ratio between hip circumference and waist circumference. This proportion is another good indicator of obesity and risk for diseases associated with metabolic syndrome.

To determine hip circumference, use the tape to measure the distance around the hips where they are widest. Then divide your waist size by your hip size. For example, if you have a twenty-four-inch waist and thirty-six-inch hips, divide twenty-four by thirty-six, and you will determine that you have a waist-to-hip ratio of .67. For women, a waist to hip ratio of .80 or less is safe. For men, a safe waist-to-hip ratio is .90 or less. A ratio greater than 1.0 is considered too high and puts one at risk for diseases such as diabetes, cardiovascular disease, and other ailments related to metabolic syndrome.

Body Fat Analysis

As noted, weight isn't the only factor that determines obesity. Two 200-pound men may have very different body types. One may have an athletic, lean body with 12 percent body fat. The other may have an untoned body with 30 percent body fat. The percentages are based on the weight of the fat as a proportion of the weight of the entire body. The normal range for body fat in women is 17 to 27 percent. For men the normal range is 12 to 24 percent. (Women naturally have more body fat than men, so their range is higher.)

Several tests are available to measure one's percentage of body fat.

Anthropometry

Here, calipers are used to measure the thickness of skin folds. The most precise measuring is done on several places on the body and charted. But even when those doing the measuring are careful, anthropometry is considered a rough guide at best.

Hydrodensitometry

This method of assessing body fat involves weighing an individual in a tank of water. First a weight measurement is taken outside the tank; then the individual is weighed in the tank. Bone and muscle densities are higher than that of water, and fat is less dense than water. Therefore, a person with more bone and muscle will weigh more in water than one with less bone and muscle. Once the individual is weighed, a mathematical formula is used to determine the percentage of body fat.

Though a better yardstick than anthropometry, hydrodensitometry also has its drawbacks. It is not as convenient as other methods. Also, if a person does not expel all air from his or her lungs before weighing, the measurement will give an inaccurately high estimate of fat content. Moreover, the tank water must be perfectly motionless during the measuring.

Bioelectrical Impedance Analysis (BIA)

For this form of measurement, a low-level electrical charge is used to estimate body fat. The person stands on two metal pads that are part of a device that passes a low-level electric signal through the body. The harmless charge is conducted through the body's tissues by water and fluids. The device assesses the total amount of water in the body and uses a mathematical formula to estimate the percentage of body fat. Fat tissue contains relatively little water—only 10 to 20 percent, while fat-free tissue may be as much as 75 percent water. Consequently, the bioelectrical impedance measurement is considered one of the easiest tests to perform and a good way to estimate body fat percentage.

BIA scales are currently available for home use, but consumers should beware that many of these machines produce inaccurate results. Also, because BIA results are based on total body water, results can vary according to how hydrated you are at the time of testing.

Near-Infrared Interactance (NIR)

This form of measurement uses a fiber-optic probe to measure tissue composition at various sites throughout the body. The probe is held next to various body parts, and the light it emits is reflected or absorbed, depending upon the characteristics of that area of the body. A detector on the probe then measures the intensity of the light bouncing off the area and uses the figure to compute body fat percentages. The NIR signal can go down only so far in the body, and much depends on the expertise of the person doing the measuring, so the process is still considered an uncertain method of determining body fat.

Dual Energy X-Ray Absorptiometry (DEXA)

Currently the gold standard of fat measurement, DEXA uses a low-dose x-ray to determine body fat percentage. The dose of radiation, according to centers that use DEXA, is lower than what a person would get on an average sunny day, and the procedure—which takes about seven minutes—is done fully clothed. It's extremely precise and safe, but it's only now making its way out of the lab and into general practice.

Diagnosing: Cholesterol Abnormalities

Testing cholesterol levels provides an indication of your risk for cardiovascular disease, including heart attack and stroke. A blood test detects cholesterol abnormalities. Because the test is checking your blood fats, or lipids, your doctor may refer to the test results as a *lipid profile.*

As the nature of cholesterol and blood lipid testing has become more advanced, physicians are able to routinely use one sample of blood to obtain a profile that provides a measurement of all cholesterol levels—total cholesterol, HDL, LDL, and triglycerides, along with various subtypes of LDL and HDL cholesterol.

Before your Cholesterol Test

So that your physician will obtain the most accurate information, you should do the following:

- Fast for twelve to fourteen hours. You are permitted to drink water, however, prior to the test.
- Do not drink alcohol for twenty-four hours prior to the test. The presence of alcohol in the system can affect test results.

- Wait six weeks after an illness. Illness may change such things as hormone balance and white blood cell counts, which could alter the composition of blood fats.
- Do not exercise twelve hours before the test. Exercise boosts HDL levels, which can give an incorrect indication of their "natural" levels.

Several medications can affect cholesterol and other blood lipids, raising their levels and changing the body's production of lipid-influencing hormones. Consult with your physician if you're taking any of the following:

- Corticosteroids
- Estrogens, such as birth control pills or hormone replacement therapy
- Testosterone replacement therapy
- Diuretics
- Psychiatric medications
- Niacin (vitamin B_3, also known as nicotinic acid)
- Various antibiotics

Some of these medications may not affect your test results, and you may be told to continue taking them as prescribed. Your doctor will likely have a record of drugs you are taking or will ask you about your medications.

Cholesterol Test Procedure

Testing for cholesterol levels involves a blood test, and it is quick and easy. The procedure can be done in a doctor's office, a lab facility, or any location with the proper staff and equipment.

When your blood is being drawn, it's always a good idea to be sitting down. This makes it easier for the health care worker to draw the blood, and it's safer for you—it prevents injury from falling should you feel light-headed.

A *phlebotomist*, a person who draws blood, will tie a tourniquet around your upper arm. After cleaning the skin on the crease between your forearm and biceps, the technician inserts a thin needle into a vein and draws a small amount of blood. You may feel the needle prick, but the pain is usually minimal.

Once the blood has been drawn and placed into three or four test-tube vials, it's sent to a lab. Results are usually returned in a few days.

Classification of Total Cholesterol (TC) Levels

Desirable	Less than 200 mg/dL*
Borderline high	200-239 mg/dl
High	240 and above

*Measurements are expressed in milligrams per liter of blood.

Classification of HDL Cholesterol Levels

High	60 mg/dl (desired level; higher is better)
Low	Less than 40 mg/dL

Classification of LDL Cholesterol Levels

Ideal	Less than 70 mg/dl
Normal	70-100 mg/dl
Borderline high	100-130 mg/dl
High	130-160 mg/dl
Very high	Greater than 160 mg/dL

How Often Should Cholesterol Levels Be Tested?

At the very least, once every five years. If you have a history of high cholesterol, you should have your blood tested annually. Many doctors will do a basic cholesterol test during your yearly physical. And if you don't have a yearly physical, there's no time like the present to get started. If you have a lipid abnormality, ask for your doctor's recommendation for the frequency of testing, which can be as often as every two or three months.

Testing Triglyceride Levels

Testing your triglycerides is also done through a blood test. Triglycerides are part of an overall lipoprotein profile. If your blood is being tested only for triglycerides, fasting for twelve hours prior to the test is absolutely necessary. Any type of food can elevate triglycerides. And watch what you eat, too. Eating fatty foods or drinking an excessive amount of alcohol within forty-eight hours prior to testing can affect triglyceride levels. You are allowed to drink water prior to the test.

Classification of Triglyceride Levels	
Normal	Less than 150 mg/dl
High	150-199 mg/dl
Very high	200-499 mg/dl
Extremely high	Greater than 500 mg/dl
Danger of pancreatitis	Greater than 1000 mg/dL

The Relationship between Triglycerides and HDL

Another way to determine whether you're at risk for heart disease is to look at your body's ratio of triglycerides to HDL. If your triglycerides are less than double your HDL, you're at a low risk for heart disease. When that ratio is higher—if your triglycerides are double or triple or quadruple the HDL—your likelihood of developing atherosclerosis and heart disease is greater, too. Experts note that the triglyceride/HDL ratio is an even stronger indicator of heart disease and atherosclerosis than the LDL to HDL ratio.

Testing: Blood Pressure

One of the most familiar of all medical tests, the blood pressure test is performed with a *sphygmomanometer*, a gauge commonly called a *blood pressure cuff.* A sphygmomanometer measures, in millimeters of mercury, the pressure of the compressed air in the cuff. Today gauges are often digital.

The Procedure

The cuff is placed around the upper arm and inflated, compressing the arm artery and stopping the blood flow. The air in the cuff is then released as the health professional listens with a stethoscope for blood coming through the artery. As soon as a sound is heard, he or she notes the number on the gauge. This number is the systolic pressure, the pressure of the heart pumping. Air is further released until no sound can be heard. The number on the gauge at this point is called the diastolic, or resting, pressure.

Classification of Blood Pressure Levels

Upper Number (Systolic)	*Lower Number (Diastolic)*
Normal below 120	Below 80
Pre-hypertension 120-139	80-89
Stage 1 hypertension 140-159	90-99
Stage 2 hypertension 160 and higher	100 and higher

Testing Variables

If you use a home testing machine to check your blood pressure, make sure it's been properly calibrated and you've been instructed on how to use it. It's important to use the correct cuff size. A cuff that's too small will give a false high blood pressure reading; a cuff that's too large will give a false low reading. It's a good idea to periodically check your home monitor readings against the pressure cuff used at your physician's office.

In some cases, a physician may order an ambulatory blood pressure monitoring, which involves wearing a monitor throughout the day. Ambulatory monitoring keeps track of changes in pressure and provides physicians with information that can more accurately diagnose high blood pressure.

Many medical professionals urge patients to have their blood pressure tested over time and in several locations, including environments such as the local drugstore or grocery store, or even at home, where you can use your own blood pressure cuff. By having several readings, your doctor can gain a better understanding of fluctuations in blood pressure measurements.

Related Diagnostic Testing

Testing for Inflammation

As mentioned earlier, inflammation in the lining of the blood vessels is linked to obesity (especially central obesity), insulin resistance, and cardiovascular disease. A test is available to measure this inflammation. The test examines the blood levels of a protein called *C-reactive protein (CRP).* This protein responds when the body experiences injury, infection, or inflammation. Elevated levels of this protein indicate a greater degree of inflammation, a risk factor for cardiovascular disease and heart attack.

This test derives its results from a blood sample, usually the same sample drawn for testing your lipid profile. The CRP test has been promoted as an excellent way to predict future cardiovascular events in apparently healthy individuals. CRP is so closely linked to metabolic syndrome that many have proposed that elevated CRP levels should be added to the diagnostic criteria.

Classifications for C-Reactive Protein

Low risk	Less than 1.0*
Average risk	1.0 to 3.0
High risk	Greater than 3.0

*The measurements for c-reactive protein are expressed in milligrams per liter of blood.

Testing Blood Clotting

Increased blood clotting is a component of metabolic syndrome that can worsen the chance of cardiovascular disease or a blood clot in the lungs or leg. Traditional tests for blood clotting–-known as *prothrombin time (PT)* and *partial thromboplastin time (PTT)* are not usually sensitive enough to pick up the blood-clotting abnormalities in metabolic syndrome. A test known as *plasminogen activator inhibitor-1 (PAI-1)* is now commonly used to detect increased blood-clotting risk in patients with obesity and metabolic syndrome.

Testing Homocysteine Levels

Homocysteine is an amino acid in the blood. High levels are toxic and have been linked to an increased risk of cardiovascular disease and blood clots, even among people who have normal cholesterol levels. Currently, there are no established guidelines for homocysteine testing and routine screening.

High homocysteine levels can be the result of a deficiency of vitamin B_9, folic acid. Low vitamin B_6 and B_{12} levels can also raise homocysteine levels.

In Summary

We have covered a number of diagnostic test procedures in this chapter. In brief, your physician can determine whether you have metabolic syndrome by asking about your medical history, performing a physical examination, and ordering blood tests. Typically a physician will be assessing:

- Fasting blood glucose levels
- Lipid profiles (HDL and LDL cholesterol and triglyceride levels)
- Blood pressure
- Weight and waist circumference
- Body mass index (BMI)

Perhaps you have discovered that you have metabolic syndrome or that you are at risk for it. In the chapters that follow, we'll examine what you can do to avoid or reverse metabolic syndrome.

Part II

Overcoming Metabolic Syndrome

4

Nutrition and Weight Loss: Reversing Metabolic Syndrome

The late anthropologist Margaret Mead once said, "It's easier to change a man's religion than his diet." Most of us who have ever tried to lose weight understand the truth of that statement. Millions of Americans struggle to lose weight. If you look at the bestseller lists, you'll find diet books at the top of the charts. Each one promises something new and easy, whether it be a low-carbohydrate or low-fat diet or one that comes from a celebrity's kitchen or even the Bible. Yet all too often we find we cannot sustain the latest fad diet. We lose weight but gain it back.

History suggests to us that the fad diets don't work well over the long term. The best approach is finding a food plan that you can live with. Weight loss and balanced nutrition are important keys to preventing or reversing metabolic syndrome.

Finding the Right Food Plan

There is not one specific diet for overcoming metabolic syndrome. There is no magic pill. You have heard it before, but the words are still true. In order to lose weight, you need to burn more calories than you take in. The key to weight loss is developing a healthful diet plan, along with physical activity regimen, and following it consistently.

Choose a food plan that works for you. Many weight-loss experts say never choose a food plan that you could not live with for the rest of your life. In other words, choose a balanced, nutritious diet over a fad diet that delivers quick results in the short term but fails you over time. Then, once you choose a good plan, stick to it. Stringing together days of healthful eating will deliver weight loss. You will find that every ounce of energy you put into losing weight is worth it. The benefits of losing weight are many.

Benefits of Losing Weight

If you have lost weight in the past or have spoken with others who have, you understand how weight loss can bring improved health, more energy, and a greater sense of well-being. The Endocrine Society, an international organization of endocrinologists, has researched the benefits of weight loss and reports the following:

- Weight loss reduces insulin resistance and reduces the risk of developing type 2 diabetes.
- Losing just 5 to 15 percent of total body weight can lower a person's chances for heart disease or stroke, because weight loss improves blood pressure, cholesterol levels, and triglycerides, and decreases inflammation in the body.
- A weight loss of ten to fifteen pounds reduces the chances a person will develop osteoarthritis of the knee,

a degeneration of the cartilage cushion between bones in the knee.

- Loss of 5 to 10 percent of total body weight can raise HDL.
- For every two pounds lost, LDL decreases by 1 percent.

How a Nation Became Overweight

Thousands of years ago, food was scarce. There were no supermarket shelves bursting with foodstuffs. Our ancestors were known as hunters and gatherers. If they found nuts and berries or killed some wild game, they ate. If they did not, they went hungry. In looking for food, they stayed on their toes, literally and figuratively. If they could find food only on the high branches of a tree, they climbed. If they had to chase an animal to eat, they ran. Likewise, if an animal decided that *they* were the prey, they ran some more. Exercise wasn't an option. It was necessary for survival.

Because food was not readily available, their bodies adapted—they became "programmed" to easily convert glucose to fat and store it. This was a valuable resource—when food wasn't available, the body could tap into its reserves.

Now, zoom ahead to a couple of hundred years ago. A number of innovations came along in rapid succession. The automobile, which led to the rise of the suburbs and shopping malls, changed the way we lived. We no longer needed to walk several miles a day. Now we drove. Factories produced finely milled grain. Refrigeration allowed the shipment of perishable foods across the world. As time went on, we produced more and more food products.

Today food is big business. It is attractive, relatively inexpensive, and inescapable. Dozens of times daily, we are exposed to enticing commercials on television, radio, newspapers, and on the Internet. We Americans spend nearly $1 trillion on food each year, according to the U.S. Department of Agriculture. We are spending more and eating more.

Clearly, our culture has advanced, but our bodies are still like those of our ancestors who had to hunt for food. So, when we eat more than we need, we simply store the extra calories as fat. If we look back at the evolution of our eating patterns, it seems almost predictable that we would become a nation that is overweight.

Tips for Succeeding at Weight Loss

Set Realistic Goals

Don't rush yourself. A weight loss of one or two pounds a week means you are succeeding. It may not seem like much if you are eager to shed pounds, but the lost pounds add up. Think of it this way: If you lose one pound a week, by the end of the year you'll have dropped fifty pounds. That's an enormous amount of weight.

Remember that crash diets usually result in just that…a crash. Starving yourself, cutting your caloric intake to the minimum, usually results in "falling off the wagon." Many nutrition experts say you should adopt a food plan that you can live with for the rest of your life.

Determine How Many Calories You Need

First, figure out how much weight you have to lose. Then begin with the number of calories each day it takes to maintain your present weight.

- Inactive people require 10 to 11 calories per pound. If you're a 150-pound woman and inactive, that means if your diet contains 1,500 calories per day, you will maintain your weight.
- Mildly active people, those who exercise rarely but are usually on their feet, burn about 13 calories per pound. That works out to 1,950 calories a day for a 150-pound woman.
- Active people, who do at least three thirty- to sixty-minute workouts per week, burn 15 calories per

pound daily. That's 2,250 calories daily for a 150-pound woman.

If you're obese, you likely weigh a bit more than 150 pounds. So, another formula to figure in is this: 3,500 calories equal one pound of body fat. If you can cut 250 calories a day—the equivalent of a chocolate bar—you can lose half a pound a week. Ideally, you should cut 500 to 1,000 calories a day, which can help you drop one to two pounds a week.

Balance Your Food Groups

For those with metabolic syndrome, an optimal diet would be made up of about 25 percent protein, 45 percent carbohydrate, and 30 percent fat, but exact percentages aren't critical. The fat should be primarily unsaturated, which is the more healthful kind.

Choose the Right Carbohydrates

Many processed carbohydrates contain finely milled grain. With the wheat bran and wheat germ milled out, these products have been stripped of many minerals, vitamins, and fiber. The white flour in these products is rapidly converted to sugar and causes a spike in blood sugar levels. Choose "complex carbohydrates"—like vegetables, fruits, and whole grains—which will be metabolized more slowly.

Develop Good Eating Habits

Part of eating right is developing good eating habits. That doesn't just mean eating the right foods; it means adhering to a schedule and listening to your body. Eat at set times. Don't let your body be overcome by extreme hunger or cravings. Eat breakfast, lunch, and dinner at the same time each day, and have a healthful snack at about the same time each day as well.

Choose healthful foods. Do you fill your snack times with cookies? Try fruit instead. Do you fill up on bread before a meal? Have a salad. If you're in a fast-food restaurant, order a healthful side dish instead of fries; drink water instead of soft drinks or fruit juices.

Control Portion Sizes

In this era of "supersizing," it is easy to overlook the importance of controlling the size of our food servings. Don't have a measuring cup handy? Use the "thumb and fist" method for measuring. Here's an easy guide to judging portion size.

- Thumb tip: one teaspoon, as in a serving of mayonnaise or margarine
- Thumb: one ounce, as in a piece of cheese
- Handful: one or two ounces of snack food, as in a handful of nuts
- Palm: three ounces, as in a cooked serving of meat
- Fist: one cup of cereal flakes

Control of portion sizes works in both directions. Most people who diet do not eat enough vegetables and fruits. You should work on increasing your portion sizes of those foods. When it comes to weight loss, vegetables and fruits should be consumed to excess. The more you eat, the more weight you will lose. Why? Because these miracle foods are high in nutrients, fiber, and water and low in calories. They help you feel full and satisfied without adding many extra calories. The best way to be successful losing weight is to keep yourself full of these healthy foods, so you have less room to eat higher calorie foods.

Keep a Food Diary

People who keep a daily diary of what they eat lose more weight. A diary is an effective way to become aware of what and how much you're eating. Often when we operate out of poorly established eating habits, we may take in far more calories a day than we realize.

Write down everything you eat and the approximate size of the serving. Note the times you had a meal or a snack. You can keep track of the calories, too, but if you're eating the right amounts of healthful foods, that shouldn't be necessary, at least not after the initial few days, when you've established your setup. After a week, look over your notes. Are you eating good foods? Are you varying your diet so it doesn't get boring? Are you "slipping"? If so, don't berate yourself. Pick yourself up and return to your plan.

Plan before You Shop

Don't go into a supermarket unprepared. Make a shopping list with appropriate food choices, and stick to it. You don't want to fall victim to impulse buying. Products in supermarkets are strategically arranged to maximize customer purchases. You'll notice certain products are at eye level, while others are placed on lower shelves and are not as easy to notice. Buy exactly what you need and nothing more. You'll find that not only is this good for your diet; it's also good for your wallet.

Dining Out

Going out for meals is more popular than ever in our fast-paced society, but if you're trying to lose weight, it can be a challenge. Though government regulations now require many

USDA Food Pyramid
Recommended Daily Servings

Grains:	6-9 servings
Fruits and Vegetables:	5-10 servings or more if possible
Dairy:	2-3 servings for men and 3-4 servings for women
Meats:	2-3 servings
Fats, Oils and Sweets:	use sparingly

Serving Sizes

Grains:
- 1 tortilla
- ½ cup cooked cereal, rice or pasta
- ½ starchy vegetable, such as potato
- ½ English muffin or hamburger bun
- 6 to 8 crackers
- ½ cup tofu

Fruits and vegetables:
- 1 medium-size piece of fresh fruit
- ½ cup dried fruit
- 1 cup leafy or raw vegetable
- ½ cup canned fruit or vegetable
- ½ cup cooked vegetable
- ¾ cup fruit or vegetable juice

Meat, poultry, and fish:
- 3 ounces (about the size of a deck of cards)

Dairy:
- 1 egg
- 1 cup yogurt
- ½ cup cottage cheese
- 1 cup milk
- 1 ounce or ½ cup cheese

Fats, oils, and sweets:
- 1 teaspoon margarine
- 1 teaspoon butter
- 1 teaspoon vegetable or canola oil

Other:
- 2 tablespoons peanut butter
- ½ cup cooked dry beans

For a personalized food pyramid plan, visit the Web at www.mypyramid.gov.

Sample Weight Loss Diet

Breakfast
- Egg-white omelet with vegetables; 1 cup fat-free yogurt; several servings of fresh fruit
- 1 cup fat-free cottage cheese; several servings of fresh fruit or vegetables
- 2 eggs; 2 slices of turkey bacon or soy sausage or a serving of fish/chicken; several servings of fresh fruit and/or vegetable

Lunch
- ½ sandwich with 2 oz. fat-free lunch meat; several servings of vegetables and fruits
- Several servings of low-fat vegetable soup
- 1 large salad with hard-boiled egg whites, chicken or turkey, and low-fat dressing
- 3-5 oz. of fish, chicken, or turkey; several servings of vegetables and fruits

Dinner
- 1 large salad with fat-free dressing; several servings of vegetables and fruits, and 3-5 oz. fish, chicken, or turkey or 3-5 oz. lean red meat (once a week)

Snacks (three times a day)
- Fruits
- Vegetables
- ½ serving (2-4 oz.) tuna or chicken
- 2 slices soy cheese or low-fat cheese
- ¾ cup unsweetened breakfast cereal; ½ cup skim milk
- 5 whole-grain crackers

restaurants to post the nutritional values of their menu items, this information is not always available. Here are a few things to keep in mind when dining out:

- If the restaurant has a Web site, look it over for nutritional information before you go.
- At the restaurant, eat a salad (with fat-free dressing) before your meal. The greens are full of nutrients and fiber, and the dish will limit your intake of the entrée.

- Have a side order of steamed vegetables in addition to your regular meal. The vegetables will help you fill up and eat less of the other food.
- Avoid appetizers. They're often high in calories and fat. True, that's not always the case, but you won't miss the dish—and you'll save a few dollars.
- Order sauces, butter, and dressings on the side.
- If you're having pasta, have tomato-based sauce. Tomatoes are rich in antioxidants—and not rich in the artery-clogging substances found in cream-based sauces.
- Don't eat any bread, if possible. Those slices will fill you up with calories in no time. If you're at breakfast, eat whole wheat bread or toast with no butter.
- Drink water, diet soda, or unsweetened tea. Avoid other soft drinks, beer, and other alcoholic beverages.
- Have a fruit cup for dessert.
- Substitute veggies for potatoes or fries. Potatoes are a high-starch item; French fries combine that starch with hot vegetable oil, which shoots the carb and fat counts off the scale.

Cooking at Home

At home, you have total control over your meal. Here are a few ideas to make those meals even better:

- Cut all liquid calories except skim milk. (Diet soda and other diet beverages, which have fewer than ten calories per serving, are okay.)

- Eat fruits and—especially—vegetables whenever you can; eat them before a main meal, to calm your appetite. Remember, when it comes to fruits and vegetables, "more is better!"
- Balance your meals and snacks. Include a small amount of low-fat protein with each meal and snack whenever you can.
- Add spices to your dishes. Just because your meals are good for you doesn't mean they have to be bland.
- Cut visible fat on meats and chicken.

Do a Self-Inventory

After the first few weeks, take an inventory of your weight-loss plan. How do you feel? Thanks to improved nutrition, you probably feel better, in addition to having lost weight. Are you sleeping better? Do you have more energy? If so, give yourself a pat on the back.

The Glycemic Index

If you have insulin resistance, the glycemic index is a valuable tool in helping to avoid spikes in blood sugar levels. The index was created in 1981 by David Jenkins, M.D. and Thomas M.S. Wolever, M.D. The two doctors noted that not all carbohydrate foods break down the same way, meaning that not all foods release glucose into the bloodstream at the same rate.

Foods with a higher glycemic index dump sugars into the bloodstream, producing an insulin spike. Foods with a lower glycemic index break down slowly and release glucose gradually into the bloodstream, keeping sugar levels more stable so that

Recommended Foods

Chicken and poultry: It's high in protein and B vitamins. Chicken and turkey are good choices. Avoid the skin, which is full of fat.

Beef and pork: These meats are high in protein, B vitamins, and stearic acid, a saturated fatty acid, which does not raise cholesterol. Choose lean cuts—the less fat, the better.

Fish: Choose cold-water fish, such as halibut and salmon, which are high in protein and omega-3 fats.

Beans: They are high in fiber and full of protein. Kidney beans and soybeans are good choices. Soybeans come in many forms, from soy milk to tofu.

Olive and canola oils: These are monounsaturated fats and contain omega-3 fats. They are still fats, however, so watch portion sizes.

Nuts: They contain monounsaturated fats, minerals, fiber, and omega-3 fats. Almonds and walnuts are good choices. Although healthy, nuts are also very high in calories, and you should have only very small portions of them. Peanut butter, which is extremely high in calories and fat, should be avoided altogether.

Fruits and vegetables: If there is a so-called miracle food for weight loss, this is it. Fruits and vegetables are high in nutrients and fiber and help you feel full. Fresh fruits and vegetables are best, but frozen and canned can also be good. Avoid dried fruits and fruit juices.

Whole grains: Grains are excellent sources of fiber, vitamin E, and minerals. Avoid processed, finely milled grains when possible. True whole-grain products are "crunchier" and will be digested more slowly.

Dairy: Milk and other dairy products contain calcium, which is good for bones and for lowering blood pressure; they also contain vitamins A and D. Choose low-fat or fat-free varieties. Use cheese in limited amounts.

Recommended Foods (continued)

Fats: The so-called good fats include *monounsaturated fats*, which remain liquid at very low temperatures. They're generally found in oils such as olive oil, peanut oil, and canola oil.

Polyunsaturated fats: Remain liquid at room temperature. They're found in oils such as corn oil, safflower oil, and soybean oil. They're also found in fish and fish oil.

Green tea: This beverage contains antioxidants, compounds that protect against cell damage inflicted by molecules called oxygen-free radicals, which are a major cause of disease and aging. Green tea is also believed to lower LDL and triglycerides. Some experts believe that green tea also has an appetite suppressing effect.

Red wine: This has been proven to lower cholesterol; however, use it in moderation—alcohol is high in calories and can raise triglycerides and blood sugar levels.

insulin does not spike. The higher the glycemic index, the greater the glucose and insulin response.

Understandably, individuals with metabolic syndrome benefit from eating foods with a lower glycemic index. Pure glucose is set at a value of 100, which happens to be the same as white bread. It is recommended that you choose foods with a low glycemic index as often as possible.

Although important, the glycemic index does not tell the whole story about the impact of glucose in the bloodstream. In 1997, Harvard University researchers introduced the concept of the *glycemic load*, which takes into account the volume of and fiber in a food item. Foods with higher fiber do not quickly flood the bloodstream with glucose. Why not? When fiber is ingested, it makes you feel full—it makes the stomach swell. This fiber slows gastric emptying, keeping the food in the stomach longer. As a result, blood sugar levels are lower and insulin does not spike.

Here's an example. Cantaloupe may have a high glycemic index (64) but a low glycemic load (4); it contains sugar, but the fiber allows the sugars to be released more slowly. Foods that have a glycemic load of 10 are considered better carbohydrates for people with metabolic syndrome.

The glycemic load is obtained by dividing the glycemic index value by 100 and then multiplying that sum by the number of grams of carbohydrate in the serving. The lower a food's glycemic load, the better it is for people with insulin resistance.

Glycemic Index Classifications

Low glycemic index	Below 55
Moderate glycemic index	56-69
High glycemic index	Above 70

Foods to Avoid

Fatty meats: These meats are usually mass-produced and heavily processed; many red meats contain high amounts of saturated fat.

Fruit juices and dried fruits: These are often high in sugar and high in calories. Fresh or frozen fruit is better.

Soft drinks and energy drinks: Avoid full-sugar drinks. They will spike blood sugar and are full of empty calories.

Beer and other alcoholic beverages: These are high in calories.

Processed carbohydrates: These foods include white bread, mashed potatoes, white rice, pasta, and most snack foods.

Salt: When you ingest salt, the body draws more water into the cells to dilute it. More fluid in the blood means the heart has to work harder and blood pressure may increase on the walls of your blood vessels.

Fats: The "bad fats" include *saturated fats*, which are solid or almost solid at room temperature. They are found in animal fats, whole-milk products, coconut oil and palm oil. Saturated fats are generally bad for you. They raise LDL cholesterol and triglycerides. *Trans fats* are even worse than saturated fats. Trans fats are produced when food manufacturers infuse hydrogen gas into oil to convert it to a solid state in order to extend the shelf life of food products. This process is called *hydrogenation*. Examples of products containing trans fats are margarine, shortening, snack foods, commercial baked goods, and commercially fried foods such as French fries. Avoid all trans fats. They raise LDL and triglyceride levels and lower HDL.

Glycemic Load Classifications

Low glycemic load	Below 10
Intermediate glycemic load	11-20
High glycemic load	Over 20

Find Support

Losing weight is often difficult to do all alone. Give yourself the benefit of support. That means emotional support and educational support. You will find emotional support especially helpful if your emotions are one reason you overeat. Educational support means learning about good nutrition and ways to avoid the disease risks that come with metabolic syndrome.

Weight-loss programs, such as Weight Watchers, can be invaluable in urging you on. Also, working with a dietitian can be most helpful; a dietitian can be supportive, help you stay accountable to yourself, and help you continually shape your diet when you feel like you're getting into a rut. Remember, the goal isn't only to lose weight; it's to build a better, healthier life.

Glycemic Food Index and Loads

	Glycemic Index	Glycemic Load
Breads		
Bagel, white, frozen	72	25
Baguette, white, frozen	95	15
Bread stuffing	74	16
Barley kernel bread, 50% barley flour	46	9
Barley flour bread, 100% barley flour	67	9
Coarse whole wheat bread	52	10
Hamburger bun	61	9
Melba toast	70	16
Gluten-free white bread (gluten-free wheat starch)	76	11
Oat bran bread	47	9
Rye kernel (pumpernickel) bread	50	6
Wholemeal rye bread	58	8
White wheat flour bread	70	10
Pita Bread	57	10
Crackers		
Breton wheat crackers	64	10
Puffed rice cakes	78	17
Rye crackers	64	11
Stoned wheat crackers	67	12
Soda crackers	74	12
Breakfast Cereals		
All-Bran	42	9
Bran Buds	58	7
Bran Flakes	74	13
Cheerios	74	15
XXX Bran	75	15

	Glycemic Index	Glycemic Load
Breakfast Cereals (continued)		
Corn Flakes	81	21
Cream of Wheat	66	17
Golden Grahams	71	18
Grapenuts	71	15
Mini Wheats, whole wheat	58	12
Muesli	49	10
Nutrigrain	66	10
Oat Bran	67	9
Quick Oats	66	17
Puffed Wheat	67	13
Raisin Bran	61	12
Rice Krispies	82	21
Shredded Wheat	75	15
Total	76	13
Wheat biscuits (plain flaked wheat)	70	13
Cereal Grains		
Pearl Barley	25	7
Buckwheat	54	16
Cornmeal	69	9
Sweet corn	53	17
Couscous	65	23
Millet	71	25
Rice, white	64	23
Rice, brown	55	18
Instant, puffed rice	69	29
Pastas		
Fettuccine	40	18
Linguine	46	22
Mung bean noodles	33	15
Macaroni	47	23

	Glycemic Index	Glycemic Load
Pastas continued		
Spaghetti, white, boiled	42	20
Vermicelli, white boiled	35	16
Fruits		
Apples, raw	38	6
Apple juice	41	11
Apricots, raw	57	5
Apricots, canned in light syrup	64	12
Apricots, dried	30	16
Banana, raw	51	13
Cherries, raw	22	3
Cranberry juice	68	16
Dates, dried	103	42
Figs, dried	61	16
Grapefruit juice, unsweetened	48	9
Grapes, raw	59	11
Kiwi fruit, raw	53	6
Lychee, canned in syrup and drained	79	16
Mango, raw	51	8
Oranges, raw	42	5
Orange juice	52	12
Paw paw/Papaya, raw	59	7
Peaches	42	5
Pears	38	4
Pineapple	59	7
Pineapple juice, unsweetened	46	15
Plums	39	5
Prunes, pitted	29	10
Raisins	64	28
Cantaloupe	65	4

	Glycemic Index	Glycemic Load
Fruits (continued)		
Strawberries	40	1
Tomato juice	38	4
Watermelon, raw	72	4
Vegetables		
Green peas	54	4
Pumpkin	75	3
Sweet corn	62	11
Carrots	47	3
Parsnips	97	12
Boiled potato	50	14
French fries	75	22
Mashed potato	91	18
Sweet potato	61	17
Tapioca	70	12
Taro	55	4
Yam	37	13
Legumes		
Baked beans	48	7
Beans, dried, boiled	29	9
Blackeyed peas	42	13
Butter beans	31	6
Chickpeas (Garbanzo beans, Bengal gram), boiled	28	8
Navy beans	38	12
Kidney beans	28	7
Lentils	29	5
Lima beans	32	10
Mung beans	31	5
Peas, dried, boiled	22	2

	Glycemic Index	Glycemic Load
Legumes (continued)		
Pinto beans	39	10
Soybeans	18	1
Split peas	32	6
Beverages		
Cola	58	15
Apple juice	40	12
Carrot juice	43	11
Cranberry juice cocktail	56	16
Grapefruit juice, unsweetened	48	11
Orange juice	50	13
Pineapple juice, unsweetened	46	16
Tomato juice	38	4
Sport Drinks	78	12
Hot chocolate mix	51	11
Water	0	0
Dairy Products		
Custard	38	6
Ice cream, regular	61	8
Ice cream, reduced or low-fat	39	5
Ice cream, premium	38	3
Milk, full fat	27	3
Milk, skim	32	4
Chocolate milk	34	9
Pudding	44	7
Yogurt	36	3
Yogurt, low-fat with aspartame	14	2
Nuts		
Cashews	22	3
Peanuts	14	1

5

Physical Activity: Why It's So Important

Physical activity is crucial to overcoming metabolic syndrome. Combined with the proper diet, physical activity can help to reduce the effects of or even eliminate the disorders that make up metabolic syndrome. However, just as it can be difficult to establish a healthful food plan, it also takes a concerted effort to start a program of increased physical activity. First, if you're overweight or out of shape, physical activity can be physically challenging. Secondly, it takes effort to make physical activity a habit—to incorporate it into your daily life.

However, if you ask those who have made the change from a sedentary lifestyle to one that involves physical activity, they will tell you the effort is worth it. Indeed, the benefits of physical activity are many.

How Physical Activity Helps to Overcome Metabolic Syndrome

When it comes to reversing metabolic syndrome, exercise is one of the best "medicines." If you're not physically active now, you know it takes effort to develop a more active lifestyle.

However, to say the benefits are worthwhile is an understatement. You will reap many rewards from a good exercise plan.

Reduces Insulin Resistance

Exercise is one of the most powerful ways to alleviate insulin resistance. Exercise helps the body to use insulin more efficiently. Increased efficiency means less insulin is needed in the body. If you already have diabetes, you have probably noticed that when you exercise, your blood sugar is much lower.

Even if you're not losing weight, exercise will still reduce your resistance to insulin. When you exercise, your muscles become stronger physically as well as metabolically. Exercise promotes blood flow to the muscles, helping your body use glucose more readily.

One major clinical trial has demonstrated that exercise reduces insulin resistance. The three-year study, known as the Diabetes Prevention Trial, was published in 2002. The study evaluated diet and exercise as a means of preventing diabetes. Subjects who had been instructed in nutrition, exercised for thirty minutes five times a week. In the end, the study showed that in a large percentage of high-risk individuals, diet and exercise prevented both diabetes and metabolic syndrome.

Promotes Weight Loss

When you exercise, your energy needs increase, and your body burns fat. This also means you lose abdominal fat, a risk factor for metabolic syndrome. The body is able to function more efficiently when it is not carrying extra weight. Additional weight strains the heart and lungs as they attempt to service body tissue beyond their capacity.

Reduces Risk of Heart Disease

The U.S. Department of Health and Human Services lists physical inactivity as a major risk factor for heart disease. Studies have shown that regular physical activity can reduce your chances of dying from heart disease by as much as 45 percent. Your heart is a muscle, and regular, consistent exercise is just as important for this muscle as for any other muscle in your body.

Exercise helps prevent heart attacks and strokes because it reverses many of the harmful conditions that cause these ailments. As we've discussed in earlier chapters, insulin resistance and elevated blood sugar and blood pressure are major risk factors for heart disease. Exercise not only lowers blood sugar and blood pressure but reduces "inflammation" in blood vessel walls, makes blood less likely to clot, and actually improves the way blood vessels function.

In fitness lingo, cardiovascular exercise is known as "aerobic exercise," or that which works the heart and lungs. This type of exercise improves the efficiency of your heart and blood vessels (cardiovascular system). With regular aerobic exercise, your heart will become stronger and more efficient and will pump more blood out with each beat. Walking, swimming, jogging, participating in aerobic exercise classes, and cycling are examples of aerobic exercise.

Improves Respiratory System

What do you need when you exercise? More oxygen. What does this mean? It means the more you exercise, the more you use your lungs. The more you use your lungs, the better they are able to absorb oxygen and to get rid of waste products.

Lungs with increased capacity help in the fight to prevent heart disease. Decreased lung capacity puts more strain on the heart, making it pump harder. Over an extended period of time, the heart muscle can become overworked, leading to a heart attack.

On the other hand, increased lung capacity allows the heart to work at a normal rate, with no strain. It has been shown that people who exercise regularly can actually increase the strength of their circulatory system, with open veins and arteries.

Lowers Blood Pressure

Physical activity can help lower your blood pressure. One reason is that when you alleviate insulin resistance, blood pressure drops. In addition, if you are aerobically fit, your heart pumps efficiently, your blood is loaded with oxygen, and your muscles are able to use oxygen and make energy. Your heart and lungs can do more work with less effort and less strain. This results in lowered blood pressure and reduced insulin resistance.

In general, you can expect your blood pressure to drop about 10 percent with exercise. The effects can be seen after as little as three weeks of regular exercise. For some people, a 10 percent drop isn't enough to make their blood pressure "normal," but for others, this is enough to keep them from needing blood pressure medications. And because exercise helps you lose weight, the blood pressure will continue to fall over time.

Improves Cholesterol Levels

Exercise has been show to increase levels of HDL (good) cholesterol and lower levels of LDL (bad) cholesterol. This beneficial effect on blood fats helps keep arteries free of blockages and helps prevent heart attacks and strokes.

Improves Flexibility

If muscles and joints aren't exercised, they become tight. If you are flexible, you may be able to prevent some common injuries and reduce lower-back and shoulder and neck pain. This should make you feel better about performing everyday jobs, and you'll continue to exercise.

Increases Muscle Endurance and Prevents Injury

The more you use your muscles, the longer they will be able to work for you. Stronger muscles are more sensitive to insulin. Exercise increases muscle mass and helps muscles become stronger, firmer, and toned. When starting an exercise program, some people find they can walk for only ten to twelve minutes without developing muscle aches. After several weeks of regular walking, they find their muscles have becoming stronger, and they can walk comfortably for longer periods of time.

Exercise helps you to prevent injury in your everyday life. Strong muscles that can work for extended periods of time without being strained will help you get through vacuuming the rug or carrying laundry up stairs. Many daily activities can be counted as physical activity. You'll find toting groceries or working in the garden less of a chore without muscle strains and back, neck, and leg pain.

Physical activity, done properly, also can help strengthen some body parts, making them less susceptible to injury during and after a workout.

Psychological Benefits of Exercising

Increased Sense of Well Being

When you exercise, your body releases endorphins, chemicals that produce feelings of happiness and well-being. Exercise is well known to reduce the symptoms of anxiety and depression and improve and enhance your mood. In fact, exercise can be as powerful as prescription antidepressants in its ability to alleviate depression.

When you exercise regularly, your lungs become more efficient. More efficient lungs take in more oxygen. Oxygen activates endorphins. In addition to giving you a sense of well-being, endorphins function as a natural appetite suppressant. So, as you exercise, you can burn calories and lose weight and feel good without an increase in appetite.

Reduces Stress

Stress magnifies insulin resistance and aggravates other components of metabolic syndrome. Exercise alleviates stress and lowers stress hormones. People who exercise regularly say they are better able to handle stress and tension. They say they feel less tired, which makes it easier to cope with everyday tensions. There is a strong connection between body and mind.

Having a regular physical routine can lead to mental fitness, as well as helping to hold off some diseases and conditions. As you continue your exercise routine, you'll have more energy, be better able to handle stress, and feel good about yourself.

Setting Up an Exercise Program

You'll need to think about your fitness goals, the types of exercise you can do or would like to learn, your budget constraints, and how much time you'll be able to allocate. Be certain to consult your physician about exercise programs that are right for you.

Before you can do it, you need to plan it. Planning exercise goals means figuring out reasonable short- and long-term goals and what the obstacles could be to these goals. While you're planning, be sure to consider your current physical condition—age, current level of fitness, and any physical injuries. For example, do you have a knee problem? If so, jogging may not be a good choice for you. However, biking or swimming could be. Write down your goals so you can remind yourself what they are from time to time.

Aerobic exercises that condition the heart and lungs include such activities as dancing, bicycling, cross-country skiing, uphill hiking, ice hockey, jogging, jumping rope, rowing, running in place, and stair-climbing. More moderate aerobic exercises include downhill skiing, basketball, field hockey, calisthenics, handball, racquetball, soccer, squash, and tennis. Higher-intensity activities—such as swimming, cycling, and running—will help build endurance and will also help to strengthen muscles.

Is it safe for you to exercise? Metabolic syndrome puts you at risk for a heart attack, and beginning a new exercise program can be physically strenuous. Most doctors recommend that patients with metabolic syndrome have a treadmill stress test, to gauge the strength of your heart, before beginning a vigorous exercise program. The American College of Sports Medicine guidelines recommend treadmill stress testing if you are over the age of forty-five or if you are over age thirty-five and have risk factors for heart disease, including high blood pressure, diabetes, high cholesterol, a family history of heart disease, or a currently inactive lifestyle.

Setting Realistic Goals

We all tend to do a bit of dreaming when we're goal setting. That's natural. The reality is, though, that what you'd like to do and what you may be able to do may have to be scrunched a little to make them agree. Identifying obstacles to your goals and coming up with a plan B will make your goals that much easier to achieve.

For example, you may decide that your fitness goal of increasing flexibility can be met by attending two-hour sunrise yoga classes four times a week. Sounds good, but be realistic. Are you really going to make it to the class four mornings a week before work? Do you think you'll really enjoy a two-hour class that starts at five in the morning and leaves you thirty minutes to shower, change, and get to work? If the answer is yes, then go for it. If the answer is probably not, then think through plan B. Perhaps there are after-work classes that fit the bill. Perhaps you can take a class or continue flexibility training on your own with videotapes or DVDs. There are always ways to accomplish realistic goals.

A well-thought-out plan is helpful. A well-thought-out plan that you can achieve is even better. So, set your fitness goals, check them out with a health care professional, and then start working toward them. You may have to try out an exercise class or two, convince the family you are serious about having an hour of private time, or tweak your goals until the schedule and the workout are happening for you. Assess your goals periodically. You'll be amazed at what you are accomplishing.

Exercise Recommendations

For most healthy people, the American Heart Association recommends exercise that will provide benefits to the heart, lungs, and circulation. That involves performing any moderate- to vigorous-intensity aerobic activity for at least thirty minutes on most days of the week at 50 to 75 percent of your maximum heart rate, the greatest number of times per minute the heart is capable of beating. You can accumulate thirty minutes in ten or fifteen-minute sessions throughout the day. What's important is to include physical activity as part of a regular routine.

These activities are especially beneficial when done regularly:

- Brisk walking, hiking, stair-climbing, aerobic exercise
- Jogging, running, bicycling, rowing, and swimming
- Activities—such as soccer and basketball—that include continuous running

If you're physically active regularly for longer periods or at greater intensity, you're likely to benefit more. But don't overdo it. Too much exercise can give you sore muscles and increase the risk of injury.

Here are some tips to help you build physical activity into your daily routine:

- Have a plan. Put your exercise in your planner or handheld device like any other appointment.

- Put on your exercise clothes first thing in the morning. If you are not wearing your street clothes, you are much more likely to get some exercise.
- Make plans with a friend to exercise.
- Park your car as far away as possible, and walk to work or the store.
- Take the stairs instead of the elevator.
- Squeeze a tennis ball to help strengthen your hands and wrists.
- Get up and walk around when you are talking on the telephone.
- Throw away the remote control.
- Tap your feet up and down while you are seated at your desk.
- Take five-minute walk breaks several times during the day.
- Play sports instead of watching sports.
- Walk during some or all of your lunch break.
- Get up early and take a walk before going to work.
- Go walk at the mall.
- Go dancing.
- Take the dog for a walk.
- Take the baby for a stroll.
- Mow the lawn.
- Turn off the TV.
- When traveling for work, use the fitness room in your hotel.

Remember, start slow. You can build up by increasing either the duration or the intensity of the workout.

Burning Calories

How many calories do you burn when you exercise? Everything you do burns calories. Even sleeping burns calories. The more intense the exercise, the more calories you burn. The other factor that affects how many calories you burn with exercise is how much you weigh. The more you weigh, the more calories you burn.

The following are calories burned for a 160-pound individual:

Low-intensity exercise: 2 calories per minute. Raking, badminton, baseball, bowling, croquet, gardening, golf, housework, Ping-Pong, shuffleboard, gardening, recreational sports, golf, weight lifting

Medium-intensity exercise: 5 calories per minute. Brisk walking, football, doubles tennis, leisurely biking, skating, sexual intimacy, downhill skiing, basketball, field hockey, calisthenics, handball, racquetball, soccer, squash, volleyball

High-intensity exercise: 11 calories per minute. Jogging, cycling, racquetball, singles tennis, swimming

Very high-intensity exercise: 18 calories per minute. Running, aerobic dancing, cross-country skiing, uphill hiking, ice hockey, jumping rope, rowing

Don't get pulled into thinking that all exercise should be high-intensity activity. Even moderate-intensity activities, when performed daily, can have long-term health benefits. They help lower the risk of cardiovascular diseases. Here are some examples: gardening and yard work, housework, dancing, playing Frisbee, playing catch with the dog, horseback riding.

Walking: Always Good Exercise

You can always take a walk. It's cheap. It's easy. And it's good for you. The President's Council on Physical Fitness (PCOPF) calls walking the most popular form of exercise. It may not get the attention of other physical activities, but walking is an exercise that is amazingly good for you.

Walking is good for everyone. When it comes to participants, according to PCOPF, it's the only exercise activity that doesn't exclude people as they get older. In fact, the highest number of regular walkers, according to a recent study, was men over sixty-five.

Planning Your Walk

So how much walking should you do? To get the benefits of walking, you just need to start, but here are some comparisons from PCOPF. You'll burn about the same number of calories walking as you would running a mile. It's also easier on your joints. And here's one of those times that being heavier pays off. Heavier people burn more calories walking the same distance than do lighter people.

Don't forget to warm up and cool down and to stretch both before and after walking. Many fitness trainers and health care professionals recommend that you try to work your way up to about forty-five minutes three to four times a week. That should be the goal, not something you do right away. Shorter distances and less time are the watchwords when you're starting out.

There are some things you should be careful about with your walking program. A good pair of shoes that provide a lot of support and have nonskid soles are very important. In addition to good shoes, you should:

- Dress appropriately for the time of year, in layers so you can shed layers if you get too warm.
- Walk in daylight or well-lit areas at night.
- Wear reflective clothes if you do walk at night.
- Walk with someone else.
- Don't wear headphones that block all outdoor sounds. It could prevent you from hearing a car.

Walking is a simple way to exercise that doesn't require a lot of equipment or a special place. You can keep up your walking program even when you are traveling. Just plan to walk on a regular basis and be flexible about your walks. If it's raining, too hot, or too cold, you don't need to skip your walk today—walk indoors.

Should You Join a Fitness Program?

This is another option. Fitness programs are offered in a wide variety of locations. Many private and public corporations have wellness centers for their employees. Have you investigated whether your employer offers such programs? A professional trainer might offer exercise and stress-reduction classes and design fitness programs; some trainers coordinate the services of other professionals, such as dietitians and massage therapists. Public school systems and municipal recreation departments sometimes hire fitness professionals to design and implement general recreation programs, adaptive programs for special needs populations, and social and organized sports activities. Check with your local community center.

When you're on vacation, you'll find fitness trainers conducting group and individual sessions, leading fitness "tours," and designing fitness programs for hotels, spas, cruise ships, and resorts.

There are many different fitness clubs to suit many different needs. If you do some exercise shopping, you'll probably find golf and tennis clubs, country clubs with swimming and exercise facilities, general health clubs, special-needs clubs (such as adaptive swimming for the physically impaired), and walking and cycling clubs in your area. So, let your fingers do the walking first and locate an exercise program that fits your needs and your schedule.

Keys to Exercise Success

- Establish short- and long-term fitness goals.
- Choose activities that you enjoy.
- Choose convenient workout locations.
- Have a regularly scheduled time to exercise.
- Keep your enthusiasm and motivation up: read articles about your chosen exercise, hang out with people who do the same exercises, exercise with a friend, etc.
- Adjust your goals and routine to suit your schedule and your body's needs.
- Keep an exercise journal that charts your progress.

Share your journal with your physician and use it as a gauge of your strengths.

Make Exercise Part of Your Lifestyle

Consider what will work for you over the years. Fitness is not a sometimes thing; it's an all-the-time thing. You decide what will work for you and what you will be able to stay with over the years. Be realistic, and start slowly and surely. Here are some tips for you to consider:

- *Get a checkup.* Speak with your physician about your plans to launch into a fitness program. You can discuss the types and lengths of exercise appropriate for you.
- *Rest and relaxation.* Rest is as important to fitness as are exercise and healthful eating. Without sufficient rest, you will lack the energy to exercise or otherwise take good care of yourself.
- *Get enough sleep.* Using the old "I'll sleep on my day off" won't work. Many studies have shown that there is no way to "catch up" on sleep. The best way to guarantee that you get all the benefits from your sleep time is to keep as regular a schedule as possible, going to sleep and waking up at the same time each day. Remember that sleep is tied to particular hormones in your body that ebb and flow at certain times of the day and night.
- *Stress reduction.* We all agree that stress is physically and mentally damaging. If you're stressed, you won't sleep well. If you don't sleep well, you won't benefit from exercise. If you don't exercise, then you won't feel well. It all fits together.

Fitness Myths : What Do You Think?

Urban myths, superstitions, and just generally incorrect information abound about exercise. Faulty information about fitness might prevent you from doing certain exercises. The following true-false quiz will help you separate exercise fact from fiction.

True or False. As you get older, you lose muscle and gain fat, no matter how active you are.

False. Most people do lose muscle mass as they age, but it has nothing to do with aging. Muscle mass has to do with one's level of physical activity, and most people become less active as they age. As a result, they have less muscle mass. But studies have shown that people who maintain the same level of physical activity as they age do not lose muscle mass. It's also commonly thought that you need fewer calories as you age. However, you need fewer calories only if you lose muscle mass. Those who maintain their muscle mass do not need fewer calories.

True or False. The more you exercise, the more protein you need.

False. Your body uses carbohydrates, protein, and fats for different types of energy. Protein is usually saved for repair (for cuts, burns, tears, etc.) and for maintaining tissues. A balanced diet will give your body the correct fuel it needs to exercise at maximum efficiency. And by the way, eating more protein does not help to build muscles.

True or False. A doctor or health care professional should check me out before I start a fitness routine.

True. A solid fitness routine requires a decent amount of planning. Part of the plan should be to get a checkup. You can have a treadmill stress test, to determine your cardiovascular fitness, or a body fat percentage test, to see where you're starting from. Many health care professionals can help you determine the types and duration of exercise best suited for you. Do your own research and also take advantage of a health care professional's expertise.

True or False. No pain, no gain.

False. It's okay to feel a little bit of the burn, but hurt is never a good thing. An occasional sore muscle or a little tenderness here or there may be part of starting a fitness program or trying out a new exercise. But "working through the pain" is bogus advice. If your brain is telling you that the leg lift hurts, it's time to stop. If an exercise is painful, it could be you're not warming up enough or not using the correct technique. Or it could be that your body is not suited for that particular type of exercise or length of workout. Pain means stop. Soreness means let your body recover and reexamine your workout.

True or False. Drinking water while you're exercising is a good idea.

True. Before, during, and after is a good idea. When you exercise, your muscles generate heat. Water helps keep the body cool so you don't overheat. Remember that 60 to 70 percent of your body is composed of water. If you don't replace the water you lose during exercise, you can become dehydrated. Dehydration can lead to confusion, fatigue, dizziness, and an irregular heartbeat.

*True or False***.** I never get thirsty when I exercise, so I must not need any water.

False. Thirst is a very poor indicator of dehydration. By the time you feel thirsty, you're probably already on the road to dehydration. During exercise, drink water early, and drink water often.

*True or False***.** If I want to lose weight, I should cut out all starchy food.

False. Carbohydrates ("starchy" food, such as pasta, rice, beans, whole wheat bread, potatoes) and proteins both have four calories per gram. No point in eliminating either. Many times, it's not the carbohydrate; it's the fat we add to the carbohydrate. Baked potatoes are not grown with sour cream, shredded cheddar cheese, and butter! Your body requires carbohydrates for fuel and does not work efficiently without sufficient amounts. It's never a good idea to eliminate an entire category of food.

*True or False***.** I have joint pain, especially in my ankles, so I can't work out.

False. Fitness training helps to improve joint flexibility, increase blood circulation, and keeps the joints mobile. There's an exercise for everyone! Consult a health care professional and devise a workout plan that will work for you without pain.

*True or False***.** Warming up is for wimps.

False. Soft tissue injuries are no fun for anyone. There are different ways to warm up, and a warmup should be a part of every exercise routine. Warm muscles are more flexible, making them less prone to injury.

True or False. I can work out any time of the day and get the same exercise benefit.

True. Some people believe that if you don't exercise in the morning, you won't get any benefit. Not so! The best time to work out is the time you've got. One tip: a good workout gives an energy boost, so you might not want to work out too close to bedtime.

A Closing Word

Given human nature, it often takes us a while to break old habits and create new ones. This seems especially true of starting an ongoing exercise regimen. Just as you might find support for a weight-loss plan, consider finding support for developing an exercise program. For example, you might find a walking buddy, a walking group, a biking group, or other such groups involved in ongoing exercise routines. Nowadays personal trainers are also available. Whatever direction you go, you will find that the payoff is immense for regular exercising.

6

Medications and Supplements: How Can They Help?

There is no question about it. America has become a "pill society." We are accustomed to taking a pill for what ails us. The most recent statistics bear this out. Americans spend $132 billion a year on drugs. That amounts to about 3 billion prescriptions from retail pharmacies annually.

For now, the best way to fight metabolic syndrome is through improving lifestyle with better nutrition and increased physical activity. Still, a variety of drugs are available to treat the manifestations and complications of metabolic syndrome. In this chapter, we'll examine the medications and supplements available to treat the disorders and complications of metabolic syndrome.

Drug Therapy: An Overview

There is no "one size fits all" when it comes to medication regimens. A drug that treats one component of metabolic syndrome may worsen another component. The goal of a treating physician is to achieve a balance between the benefits of a medication and the risk of possible side effects. The overall goals of drug treatment are to control or manage the following:

- *Cardiovascular disease.* Preventing or treating cardiovascular disease (heart attacks and strokes) is the ultimate goal of treating any of the disorders of metabolic syndrome.
- *Insulin resistance.* Medications can make insulin work more efficiently, lowering blood sugar and insulin levels, reducing the risk of diabetes.
- *Lipid abnormalities.* Medications can improve all of the lipid abnormalities associated with metabolic syndrome.
- *High blood pressure.* Blood pressure medications can either help or hurt other components of metabolic syndrome.
- *Obesity.* Many medications used to treat metabolic syndrome help with weight loss, but others may cause weight gain.
- *Blood clotting.* Medications that reduce blood clotting are used in metabolic syndrome to reduce the risk of cardiovascular disease.
- *Inflammation.* Many medications used to treat the components of metabolic syndrome work, in part, by reducing inflammation.
- *Associated hormone problems.* To adequately treat metabolic syndrome, all hormone imbalances must be addressed.

Diabetes Medications

Because insulin resistance is an underlying cause of both type 2 diabetes and metabolic syndrome, it is logical that diabetes medications are first-line treatments.

Metformin (Glucophage, Glucophage XR, and generics)

As the world's leading prescribed medication for diabetes, metformin is a medication frequently used to treat metabolic syndrome. It works by reducing the liver's natural production of sugar and by improving insulin sensitivity. Studies have shown that metformin can actually prevent metabolic syndrome in people at high risk. Metformin can lower LDL cholesterol and triglyceride levels but has minimal effect on HDL cholesterol. Metformin does help with weight loss, but improved nutrition and physical activity are necessary to see this effect. Metformin also has proven benefit in reducing the risk of cardiovascular disease. The original, short-acting version seems to work better for weight loss and for treating metabolic syndrome. The long-acting version is a specially designed pill to slowly release metformin over a day; it can be taken once a day and has fewer side effects.

Possible Side Effects

The most common side effects are nausea, diarrhea and upset stomach, which occur in about 25 percent of the people who take it. These side effects are usually temporary and subside within a couple of days, but may persist longer. To minimize side effects, start with a low dose and gradually increase it over several months. Taking metformin with a substantial meal will also reduce side effects. Metformin should not be used by people who drink heavily or have a severe infection, or have kidney or liver, disease because of a rare side effect known as lactic acidosis.

Rosiglitazone (Avandia) and Pioglitazone (Actos)

These drugs belong to a class of diabetes medications known as thiazolidinediones, or TZDs. They treat metabolic syndrome by reducing insulin resistance. These drugs make fat cells and muscle cells more sensitive to insulin by turning on and off genes in the cells. TZDs can improve many components of metabolic syndrome, including improving blood sugar levels, lowering blood pressure, and reducing inflammation and blood clotting. They decrease triglycerides and raise HDL levels and can shift LDL from the dangerous small, dense type to the less dangerous large, fluffy type. TZDs can be helpful in the treatment of cardiovascular disease and fatty liver disease. These medications redistribute body fat, moving it from dangerous areas, like the belly and vital organs, to safer areas like the hips and buttocks and under the skin.

Possible Side Effects

The most notorious side effect of TZDs is weight gain, though most people gain only a few pounds or none at all. Another side effect is fluid retention, which can result in swelling of the legs. People who have a history of heart failure can see a worsening of their condition due to the fluid retention and should not take TZDs. The lowest doses (Avandia two milligrams or Actos fifteen milligrams) seem to be best for treating metabolic syndrome without causing weight gain or fluid retention. TZDs have been criticized because they may cause a slight rise in LDL cholesterol, but this seems to be offset by improvements in LDL quality.

Metformin Combination Medications

This group includes Avandamet (rosiglitazone and metformin) and Actoplus Met (pioglitazone and metformin). Metformin and TZDs work so well together that manufacturers have combined them in one pill. These medications are ideal for treating metabolic syndrome, because of their synergistic actions. Metformin also seems to minimize the weight gain caused by TZDs. The combination pills are convenient and cut down on insurance copays, but have no additional advantages over taking the medications separately.

Exenatide (Byetta)

This is a hormonal medication that imitates the actions of a digestive hormone known as glucagon-like peptide-1 (GLP-1). It was originally derived from the saliva of the gila monster, but is now produced synthetically. It is an injection taken twice a day from a prefilled pen device. Exenatide lowers blood sugar levels, improves lipid levels, and helps with weight loss.

Possible Side Effects

Nausea is the most common side effect, because exenatide slows down the digestive system, but that effect is usually temporary. It can also interfere with the absorption of other medications, so they should be taken at least one hour before exenatide. There is also the inconvenience of taking an injection twice a day.

Pramlintide (Symlin)

Another hormonal diabetes medication, this drug works by mimicking hormones that regulate blood glucose. Pramlintide is a synthetic version of the hormone *amylin*, which, like insulin, is produced by the pancreas to help lower blood sugar. Pramlintide is not widely used to treat metabolic syndrome, but may help some people who already have diabetes. It allows patients with diabetes to lower their dose of insulin. Like exenatide, pramlintide is given as an injection.

Possible Side Effects

Some people experience nausea, vomiting, low blood sugar, or headache.

Cholesterol Medications

Statins

A class of drugs known as *statins* or *HMG-CoA reductase inhibitors* are medications commonly used to treat abnormal cholesterol levels. They are best for lowering LDL levels, but some can have a modest favorable effect on triglycerides and HDL levels. This class includes medications like *atorvastatin* (Lipitor), *pravastatin* (Pravachol), *simvistatin* (Zocor), and others that end in "statin."

These drugs work by blocking an enzyme needed to produce cholesterol. Statins not only reduce overall LDL levels but also improve the quality of LDL from the dangerous small, dense type to the less dangerous large, fluffy type. Statins also have been shown to have beneficial antioxidant effects, decreasing inflammation and blood clotting. By reducing LDL *levels* and improving LDL *quality* as well as reducing blood vessel inflammation and blood clotting, statins can dramatically reduce the occurrence of cardiovascular disease and can even reverse its progress. As research in this field continues to show dramatic long term benefits, statins are being used more and more commonly and in higher doses than ever before.

Possible Side Effects

The most common side effects of statins are liver inflammation and muscle problems that can range from mild aches and pains to severe muscle damage. The liver should be monitored with periodic blood tests and anyone on a statin drug should immediately report muscle pain or weakness to their physician. Because statins have such tremendous health benefits, many doctors will recommend that you continue taking a statin if it is causing only mild muscle pain.

Commonly Prescribed Statins

- Atorvastatin (Lipitor)
- Fluvastatin (Lescol, Lescol Xl)
- Lovastatin (Mevacor, Altoprev, and generics)
- Pravastatin (Pravachol)
- Rosuvastatin (Crestor)
- Simvastatin (Zocor)

Fibric Acid Derivatives

Also known as fibrates, this class of drugs includes fenofibrate (*Tricor, Lofibra*) and an older, less effective version known as gemfibrozil (*Lopid and generics*). Actually a distant cousin of the TZDs, fibrates are an excellent choice for metabolic syndrome because they lower triglycerides and LDL cholesterol while raising HDL cholesterol.

Possible Side Effects

Side effects are uncommon, but liver problems and muscle problems can occur.

Niacin (Niaspan)

Also known as nicotinic acid or vitamin B_3, niacin, in high doses, lowers triglycerides and LDL cholesterol while raising HDL cholesterol. Standard niacin is available as an over-the-counter supplement but can be difficult to take because the dosages needed (usually 1,000 to 2,000 milligrams per day) frequently cause side effects. To minimize side effects, a slow-release prescription formulation of niacin, known as Niaspan, has been developed.

Possible Side Effects

Niacin frequently causes flushing, warm tingling of the skin, and even a burning sensation. Side effects are lessened by starting at a low dose and gradually increasing the dose over several months. The flushing can also be reduced by taking an aspirin and drinking a full glass of water one hour before taking the niacin. Other side effects of niacin include liver problems, worsening of insulin resistance, and possible blood sugar elevations in people with diabetes. Even though niacin is available without a prescription, it should be taken only under medical supervision.

Bile Acid Sequestrants

These cholesterol-lowering drugs are also known as bile acid sequestrants because they pull cholesterol out of digestive juices (bile) and allow it to pass out in the stool. The drugs in this class include *Cholestyramine (Questran, Questran Light), Colestipol (Cholestid), and Colesevelam (WelChol).* Cholestyramine and Colestipol come in granular form, in packets or canisters, and are mixed with water. A bile acid sequestrant is usually taken several times a day. Questran Light, a sugar-free version, is recommended for people with blood sugar problems. WelChol is a tablet taken once or twice a day. Bile acid resins are good only for lowering LDL cholesterol; they can actually raise triglyceride levels.

Possible Side Effects

Constipation is a common side effect of bile acid sequestrants. This can be minimized by taking a fiber supplement and getting plenty of water to drink. Many people complain about the taste and inconvenience of the granules. To improve the taste and convenience, mix it up in advance, with 50 percent juice and 50 percent water and store it in the refrigerator.

Ezetimibe (Zetia)

This is a once-a-day pill that primarily lowers LDL cholesterol by blocking absorption of cholesterol from the intestines. Ezetimibe has minimal effect on triglycerides and HDL cholesterol.

Possible Side Effects

Side effects are unusual but include abdominal pain and diarrhea.

Omega-3 Fatty Acids (Omacor)

Omega-3 Fatty Acids have been shown to reduce triglyceride levels. These beneficial "fats" are found in cold water fish such as salmon and halibut. Nutritional supplements have been used for years as a treatment for high triglyceride levels; however, the advantage to the prescription formulation of omega-3 fatty acids, Omacor, is that it is a more pure and potent formulation since the manufacturing process is regulated by the FDA.

Possible Side Effects

Side effects include upset stomach and belching and a bad taste in the mouth.

Combination Medications

Vytorin (Combination of Ezetimibe and Simvastatin)

The two drugs work together to lower LDL cholesterol. You can get the same effect by combining ezetimibe with any of the statin medications.

Advicor (A Combination of Long-Acting Niacin and Lovastatin)

This combination of a statin and niacin is useful; however, lovastatin has more side effects than other statins. You can achieve the same results by combining Niaspan with any of the other statin medications.

Blood Pressure Medications

High blood pressure, also called hypertension, is one of the most common ailments in the United States and the industrial world. In the United States, one out of three adults is afflicted with it. It is considered a major risk factor for cardiovascular disease, and when it occurs in association with other features of metabolic syndrome, the risk goes up exponentially.

Modern medicine has devised an ever-increasing variety of drugs to treat high blood pressure. Some of these drugs are beneficial to metabolic syndrome, because they can improve insulin resistance and can reduce the risk for diabetes and cardiovascular disease. On the other hand, some drugs, although good for blood pressure, can worsen insulin resistance and slow metabolism and are not, therefore, ideal choices for people with metabolic syndrome.

ACE Inhibitors

The term "ACE" is an abbreviation for "angiotensin-converting enzyme." These drugs inhibit the production of a hormone—angiotensin—required to tighten blood vessels known as ("angio" refers to "blood vessel"; "tensin" means "to tighten"). ACE inhibitors are good at lowering blood pressure, but the benefits of this class of drugs go far beyond this effect. ACE inhibitors have proven benefits in reducing the risks of diabetes, kidney disease, and cardiovascular disease. Because of these additional benefits, ACE inhibitors are considered one of the best medications for people with metabolic syndrome. It is important to know that in order to see the protective benefits from an ACE inhibitor, the maximum dosage is usually needed (even if blood pressure can be controlled at a lower dose).

There are at least a dozen ACE inhibitors on the market. The names of all generics end in "-pril" and include rampiril, lisinopril, benazepril and quinapril.

Possible Side Effects

Dry cough, headache, fatigue, and an allergic reaction that can cause sudden trouble in swallowing or breathing are the most common side effects. ACE inhibitors also can raise potassium levels, so this should be checked with a blood test a few weeks after starting the medication. Potassium is a very significant body mineral, important to cellular function.

Angiotensin Receptor Blockers (ARBs)

ARBs are close relatives of ACE inhibitors. ARBs, angiotensin receptor blockers, block the receptor for the vessel-tightening hormone angiotensin. The effects of ARBs are similar to those of

ACE inhibitors, but these medications are much newer and have less proven benefit when it comes to prevention of diabetes or cardiovascular disease. ARBs are usually prescribed for patients who can't take ACE inhibitors. Generic names of ARBs end in "-artan" and include ibesartan (Avapro), candesartan (Adacand), losartan (Cozaar), valsartan (Diovan), and olmesartan (Benicar).

Possible Side Effects

Side effects are not common but can include an allergic reaction and an elevation of potassium levels.

Carvedilol (Coreg)

This medication is a newer version of a class of drugs known as beta-blockers, which treat high blood pressure and some other heart conditions by reducing the heart rate and the heart's output of blood. All beta blockers are good at lowering blood pressure but have side effects that include slowing of metabolism and worsening of insulin resistance. Carvedilol is a unique version called an alpha-beta blocker that can actually improve insulin resistance.

Possible Side Effects

Side effects include difficulty breathing, slow heartbeat, and fatigue.

Potassium-sparing diuretics

Generic names are spironolactone, amilioride, and triamterine. These are mild diuretics that may be helpful for metabolic syndrome in that they lower blood pressure and raise potassium levels. Potassium is important for proper insulin action, and low potassium is a cause of insulin resistance.

Possible Side Effects

Side effects can include liver problems, allergic reaction, and elevation of potassium levels. Potassium levels and liver health should be monitored at regular intervals.

Weight-Loss Medications

Weight-loss medications can be helpful for treating metabolic syndrome when combined with proper nutrition and physical activity. There are no ideal medications, however, and the effects of available medications are mild at best. Clinical trials have universally shown that patients who lose weight with a weight-loss medication almost always gain it back when the medication is discontinued.

Orlistat (Xenical)

Orlistat works as a digestion inhibitor. The medication slows or blocks the digestion of fat, causing about a third of the fat from the diet to be passed in the stool. The average weight loss seen with Orlistat is about twenty-five pounds in six months. Orlistat has proven benefits that correspond with weight loss, including lowering of blood sugar and blood pressure and improvement in lipid levels.

Possible Side Effects

The most common side effect of Orlistat is diarrhea or an oily discharge. This side effect can be minimized by eating a diet that is no more than 30 percent fat and by taking a fiber supplement. Orlistat also has the theoretical risk of blocking the absorption of certain vitamins, so it is recommended that those who use it take a standard multivitamin.

Sibutramine (Meridia)

Sibutramine is an appetite suppressant that works in the brain in a similar way to many antidepressants. It has its strongest action in increasing the feeling of satiety during a meal, meaning you feel full more quickly. The effects are mild at best, and the average weight loss with sibutramine is twenty-five pounds in six months.

Possible Side Effects

High blood pressure, rapid heartbeat, insomnia, and agitation are the most common side effects. It is recommended that you have your blood pressure monitored regularly while taking this medication. You should not take sibutramine if you have cardiovascular disease or uncontrolled blood pressure.

Rimonabant (Acomplia)

This drug is known as an *endocannabinoid receptor blocker*; it blocks the action of brain chemicals that have actions similar to marijuana (cannabis). In other words, it acts like an "anti-marijuana" drug. The drug was developed with the knowledge that marijuana smokers are known to experience extreme hunger. Rimonabant not only causes weight loss but also reverses many of the components of metabolic syndrome.

Possible Side Effects

Nausea, vomiting, and depression are potential side effects.

Antidepressants

Venlefaxine (Effexor) and Duloxitine (Cymbalta)

These antidepressant medications work to alter brain chemicals that decrease appetite—the same brain chemicals (serotonin and norepinepherine) affected by the weight-loss medication Sibutramine.

Possible Side Effects

High blood pressure, rapid heartbeat, and insomnia are potential side effects. It is recommended that you have your blood pressure monitored regularly while taking these medications.

Bupropion (Wellbutrin)

Bupropion is an antidepressant with a unique mechanism of action but seems to be as effective for weight loss as any of the weight-loss medications.

Possible Side Effects

Side effects include agitation, insomnia, and in rare cases, seizures.

Antiseizure/Antimigraine Medications

Zonisamide (Zonegran) and Topiramate (Topamax)

These drugs have been shown to help with weight loss by decreasing appetite and preventing overeating. They appear to be particularly helpful in reducing episodes of binge eating and of eating at night. Some patients have had dramatic success with these medications, but high doses are sometimes necessary to achieve appreciable weight loss.

Possible Side Effects

Tingling of the hands, sedation, and memory problems have been reported.

Aspirin

Aspirin is one of the best known medications for reducing blood clotting and preventing cardiovascular disease. For this reason, it is recommended that everyone with metabolic syndrome take a "baby" aspirin (81 milligrams) every day.

Testosterone Replacement Therapy

This therapy is for men only. Testosterone is called an "anabolic" hormone, because it builds muscle. Testosterone deficiency, known as *hypogonadism*, is extremely common in men with metabolic syndrome. Men with testosterone deficiency have less muscle, a condition that worsens insulin resistance. Testosterone replacement reverses metabolic syndrome and improves insulin sensitivity. Testosterone replacement is available as an injection, topical gel (*Androgel, Testim*), skin patch (*Androderm*), or a sustained release capsule absorbed through the gums (*Striant*).

Possible Side Effects

Acne, insomnia, and agitation have been reported. There is a theoretical risk of prostate problems as well. All men should be checked for prostate cancer before starting testosterone replacement therapy.

Vitamins, Minerals, and Supplements

People with metabolic syndrome need not rely solely on prescription medication to address the problems of the condition. There are a variety of nutritional supplements that have positive health effects. When added to a proper diet and regular exercise, these vitamins and minerals and widely available foods can help diminish some effects of metabolic syndrome.

Folic acid (Vitamin B_9)

Folic acid helps prevent heart disease by aiding in the breakdown of an unhealthy amino acid known as homocysteine. Studies have shown that having elevated homocysteine levels increases the risk for cardiovascular disease and that folic acid supplementation can lower homocysteine levels. The Centers for Disease Control and Prevention strongly encourages intake of folic acid, particularly among pregnant women, because the vitamin is believed to prevent certain birth defects, such as spina bifida.

Sources: Whole grains, green leafy vegetables, nuts, avocados, bananas and oranges. It's also often added to breads, rice, and cereals. The U.S. recommended daily allowance (RDA) for the vitamin is 400 micrograms (0.4 milligrams), but doses up to 1,000 micrograms (1 milligram) may be ideal.

Chromium

This mineral, required in trace amounts, works with insulin in assisting cells to take in glucose and release energy (that is, it improves metabolism of glucose). Chromium deficiency is a cause of insulin resistance, and correcting the deficiency improves insulin sensitivity. However, there is no proof that chromium supplementation helps people that do not have chromium deficiency, and it has not been shown to cause weight loss.

Sources: Fruit juices, molasses, beef, and hard cheeses. The government has not set an RDA standard for chromium. Chromium is also available in pill form.

Omega-3 fatty acids

Omega-3 fatty acids decrease triglycerides, lower the growth rate of arterial plaques, and lower blood pressure.

Sources: Found in cold-water fish, such as salmon, sardines, tuna, rainbow trout, anchovies, and herring. A related compound—alpha-linolenic acid—is found in tofu, flaxseed, walnuts, and other foods. The American Heart Association recommends eating fish twice a week and taking supplements that contain omega-3 fatty acids.

Niacin (vitamin B_3)

As noted in the cholesterol section, niacin is important to the digestive system, assisting in converting food to energy. It lowers triglycerides and LDL cholesterol while raising HDL cholesterol.

Sources: High-protein foods such as meat, chicken, fish, peanuts, pork, and milk.

Red Yeast Rice

Used in China for centuries as both food and medicine, this simple dish works against an enzyme called HMG-CoA reductase. This is the same enzyme that is blocked by statin drugs.

Source: Made from fermenting a kind of yeast (*Monascus purpureus*) over rice. Available as a supplement in pill form.

Garlic

This root plant has antioxidant properties, and there is some evidence it helps lower cholesterol. It also appears to work as an antibiotic.

Sources: In addition to the produce aisle of your local grocer, garlic is available in odorless, tasteless pill form for those who want to avoid garlic breath.

Policosanol

This supplement appears to raise HDL and lower LDL.

Source: A substance derived from the surface of the sugarcane plant and available as a supplement in pill form.

Soy

The soybean (or soya bean, in Asian cultures) is a rich source of several nutrients, including protein and isoflavones, which may have positive effects in humans, such as cancer inhibition, increased bone strength, and a decrease in heart disease. Isoflavones help cut LDL cholesterol, as well as being a healthy source of fiber.

Sources: Soybeans, soybean oil, tofu, and soy milk.

Guggul (Gugulipid)

Indian cultures have used this ancient herb for centuries. Not only does it raise HDL and lower LDL; it also cuts triglycerides, has antioxidant properties, and acts against blood clots.

Sources: Guggul comes from the gummy resin of the mukul myrrh tree. It's available as a supplement in pill form.

Green Tea

This ancient drink is rich in nutrients that lower LDL cholesterol levels, decrease appetite, and inhibit the abnormal formation of blood clots. Unlike herbal teas, green tea does contain caffeine.

Sources: Green tea is available in loose or tea bag form in most grocery stores.

Capsaicin

This substance—which makes hot peppers hot—has been found to boost metabolism and may lower cholesterol and blood pressure.

Sources: Available as an herbal supplement and in spicy foods such as chili peppers.

Caffeine

Caffeine stimulates metabolism and should be used in moderation. Studies have linked coffee consumption to a decrease in diabetes risk.

Sources: Coffee, green tea, and black tea.

Plant Phytosterols (Beta Sitosterol)

Phytosterols closely resemble cholesterol, and it is believed that they can actually block food-based cholesterol from being absorbed into the bloodstream. The result is that both phytosterols and dietary cholesterol end up excreted in waste matter.

Sources: Rice bran, wheat germ, corn oils, vegetable seeds, avocados, and soybeans.

Fiber

Fiber is helpful because it adds volume and bulk to food without adding calories. It helps you feel satisfied. Fiber aids in digestion and helps create a well-formed and easily passed stool.

Sources: Whole grains, legumes, fresh fruit and vegetables; over-the-counter fiber supplements such as Metamucil, Citrucel, and Benefiber.

Oat Fiber

A powerful fiber source, oats lower the risk of cardiovascular disease.

Sources: Oats are best in rawer forms, such as oat bran and steel-cut oats, and are readily available at grocery stores.

Ginseng

The species *Panax Ginseng* contains chemicals that are thought to lower blood sugar levels and improve insulin resistance.

Sources: The herb ginseng.

Fenugreek

The seeds of fenugreek, an herb, are thought to have glucose-lowering properties and to decrease appetite.

Sources: Available as a seed, as a tea, or in the form of sprouts.

Bitter Melon

This herb is widely used in Asia and South America to treat diabetes because of its ability to alleviate insulin resistance.

Sources: This vegetable is a member of the Cucurbitaceae (gourd) family and a relative of squash, watermelon, muskmelon, and cucumber.

Medications that May Aggravate Metabolic Syndrome

Some medications adversely affect metabolic syndrome. Some such drugs promote weight gain; others may lead to type 2 diabetes.

Corticosteroids

This class of drugs, used to treat conditions—such as asthma, arthritis, and lupus—works by quieting an overactive immune system. These steroids are different from anabolic steroids, which are used for androgen replacement in men or abused by bodybuilders. Corticosteroids promote fat accumulation and muscle loss and cause weight gain and severe insulin resistance. Corticosteroids can cause diabetes and can increase the risk of cardiovascular disease and other ailments. Common corticosteroids include prednisone, hydrocortisone, dexamethasone, and methylprednisolone.

Sulfonylureas

These are medications used to treat type 2 diabetes by stimulating the pancreas to produce more insulin. Ironically, in treating diabetes, they may worsen the disease by increasing insulin levels and insulin resistance. Sulfonylureas are notorious for causing weight gain. Common sulfonylureas are glyburide (DiaBeta), glipizide (Glucotrol), and glimepiride (Amaryl).

Antidepressants

Many antidepressants have weight gain as a side effect, which can worsen metabolic syndrome. This is because the same brain chemicals involved in depression help to regulate appetite centers. Older antidepressants, such as amitriptyline and nortriptyline are known to cause massive weight gain. Mirtazapine (Remeron) frequently causes weight gain as well. Other antidepressants such as fluoxetine (Prozac), sertraline (Zoloft), paroxetine (Paxil), citolopram (Celexa), and escitalopram (Lexipro) can cause some people to gain weight.

Antiseizure Medications

Although originally developed to treat epilepsy, these medications *carbamazepine (Tegretol)* and *gabapentin (Neurontin)* are being used more and more to treat other conditions, including chronic pain, migraine headaches, and diabetic nerve pain. These medications frequently cause sedation and weight gain.

Antihistamines

Older antihistamines—most notably diphenydramine (Benadryl)—can cause sedation and weight gain. Many sleeping pills, including Tylenol PM, also contain diphenhydramine.

Diuretics

The diuretics *furosemide* and *hydrochlorothiazide* cause loss of potassium in the urine, which may contribute to insulin resistance. Although sometimes necessary for adequate blood pressure control, potassium supplementation can prevent worsening of insulin resistance.

Calcium Channel Blockers

Though medications in this class are good at lowering blood pressure, they can worsen insulin resistance and can increase the risk of diabetes. Drugs include amlodipine (Norvasc), nifedipine (Procardia), verapamil (Calan), and diltiazem (Cardiazem).

Beta-Blockers

This class of blood pressure medications, once considered a top choice for blood pressure control, is not always ideal for patients with metabolic syndrome, because beta-blockers can slow metabolism and worsen insulin resistance. Drugs include propanolol (Inderal), metoprolol (Toprol), and atenolol (Tenormin).

Newer Antipsychotics

These medications—which include olanzapine (Zyprexa), risperidone (Risperdal), and quetiapine (Seroquel)—have been associated with an increased risk of dramatic weight gain, type 2 diabetes, increased LDL cholesterol, decreased HDL cholesterol, and elevated triglycerides. Research is being done to investigate the connection between these drugs and metabolic syndrome risk factors.

HIV/AIDS Medications

A class of drugs known as protease inhibitors—among them nelfinavir (Viracept), ritonavir (Norvir), saquinavir (Invirase, Fortovase), and tipranavir (Aptivus)—cause severe insulin resistance with increased belly fat, elevated blood sugar, and lipid abnormalities. Using these drugs can cause a condition known as "HIV lipodystrophy," which is similar to metabolic syndrome.

In Summary

As we've noted, a number of medications and supplements may play a helpful role in overcoming metabolic syndrome. And since metabolic syndrome includes a constellation of conditions, it's very likely that your doctor will prescribe several prescription medications. However, drugs alone will not reverse metabolic syndrome. Here are other things you can do to reverse or prevent metabolic syndrome.

- Lose weight, and maintain weight in the normal range.
- Make dietary changes. Choose a diet low in trans fats and saturated fats and high in vegetables, fruits, whole grains and healthy protein.
- Exercise at least thirty to sixty minutes a day, six days a week.
- Take medications as prescribed.
- Stop smoking.
- Drink alcohol only in moderation.
- Relax! Reduce stress.
- Get plenty of sleep.
- See your physician on a regular basis.

If you make these lifestyle changes, along with taking appropriate medications, you have a good chance at overcoming metabolic syndrome. You are already armed with a basic understanding of the syndrome and what you need to do to reverse it. Develop a plan, put it into action, and stay with it—a day at a time. Research shows that even modest weight loss and increased physical activity can produce significant gains in the way your body's metabolism works.

Resources

American Obesity Association
1250 24th Street, NW
Suite 300
Washington, DC 20037
(202) 776-7711
www.obesity.org

An organization devoted to changing perceptions about obesity, including recommending recognition of obesity as a disease, making obesity a public health priority, and advancing treatments of obesity.

American Heart Association
National Center
7272 Greenville Avenue
Dallas, TX 75231
(800) AHA-USA1 (242-8721)
www.americanheart.org

The American Heart Association offers information about cardiovascular disease and, on its Web site, has resources to "help live a longer, stronger life." A "Healthy Lifestyle" link on its Web site has suggestions for diet and nutrition, lowering cholesterol, and exercise and fitness.

American Diabetes Association
1701 North Beauregard Street
Alexandria, VA 22311
(800) DIABETES (342-2383)
www.diabetes.org

A non-profit health organization "providing diabetes research, information and advocacy." Along these lines, the American Diabetes Association funds research and offers tips on diabetes prevention. The Web site also features nutrition information and recipes.

National Center for Complementary and Alternative Medicine
National Institutes of Health
Bethesda, MD 20892
(888) 644-6226
http://nccam.nih.gov

One of many centers that fall under the aegis of the National Institutes of Health (which is, in turn, part of the Public Health Service in the Department of Health and Human Services), the NCCAM looks at alternative healing processes, which it supports with research funding, training, and integration into the mainstream medical community. Its Web site features a particularly helpful page devoted to nutritional supplements.

Overeaters Anonymous
World Service Office
PO Box 44020
Rio Rancho, NM 87174-4020
(505) 891-2664
www.oa.org

A twelve-step group that provides support for those whose goal is to overcome compulsive eating. OA includes a twelve-step program and is not just for the overweight; members include people of average or less-than-average size who share an unhealthy compulsion with weight, food, and size. The concept of abstinence from overeating is the basis of OA's program of recovery, but it encourages the use of professionals to assist with overcoming an eating fixation.

American Dietetic Association
120 South Riverside Plaza, Suite 2000
Chicago, IL 60606-6995
(800) 877-1600
www.eatright.org

The largest organization of nutrition professionals in the United States, the ADA includes registered dietitians, dietetic technicians and food-service managers and educators.

Recipelink.com
www.recipelink.com

A Web site that serves as a clearinghouse for recipes of all kinds. The diet-conscious will find recipes targeted to diabetics, those with food allergies, and people desiring low-carb and/or low-calorie meals.

Centers for Disease Control and Prevention
1600 Clifton Road
Atlanta, GA 30333
(404) 639-3311 (direct)
(404) 639-3534 (public inquiries)
(800) 311-3435
Overweight and obesity resources:
www.cdc.gov/nccdphp/dnpa/obesity/resources.htm

The CDC, a unit of the Department of Health and Human Services, has a wide-ranging portfolio that includes studying the roots of disease and protecting the health and safety of all Americans. Because obesity is a major public health concern, the CDC maintains a Web page devoted to information about the subject, including links to HHS/Department of Agriculture's 2005 dietary guidelines (which can be found at http://www.healthierus.gov/dietaryguidelines/) and a wide variety of consumer information.

National Heart, Lung and Blood Institute: Obesity Education Initiative
NHLBI Health Information Center
P.O. Box 30105
Bethesda, MD 20824-0105
(301) 592-8573
www.nhlbi.nih.gov/about/oei

The NHLBI, also part of the National Institutes of Health, focuses on diseases of the cardiovascular system and lungs, as well as sleep disorders. It began its Obesity Education Initiative in 1991 to educate the public on the problems of overweight, as well as to foster programs to combat obesity.

National Heart, Lung and Blood Institute: National Cholesterol Education Program
www.nhlbi.nih.gov/chd

Another initiative of the NHLBI, this program works to lower coronary heart disease by reducing the number of Americans with high cholesterol. September, incidentally, is National Cholesterol Education Month.

Community Nutrition Institute
419 West Broad Street #204
Falls Church, VA 22046
(703) 532-0030
www.communitynutrition.org

CNI is a national nonprofit organization, founded in 1970, which provides information, education, and training on domestic and international food and nutrition concerns. Among its projects are a focus on food and nutrition in low-income communities (which often have a disproportionately high rate of malnutrition and obesity); food safety initiatives; and environmental work.

MedlinePlus
U.S. National Library of Medicine and National Institutes of Health

U.S. National Library of Medicine

8600 Rockville Pike
Bethesda, MD 20894
http://medlineplus.gov

An Internet resource containing information about drugs and health topics, a dictionary and encyclopedia, and links to physician listings across the United States.

U.S. Department of Agriculture Food, Nutrition and Consumer Service

3101 Park Center Drive, Room 926
Alexandria, VA 22302
703-305-2281 (Communications and Government Affairs)
www.fns.usda.gov/fncs

A division of the Department of Agriculture that focuses on food safety and reducing hunger. To that end, it administers a variety of food distribution and assistance programs, with Web site links to nutrition and lifestyle tips.

Glossary

acanthosis nigricans: A skin condition caused by excess insulin, which causes patches of skin, usually on the neck, armpits, knuckles and face, to take on a black velvety appearance, as if the skin were dirty. Acanthosis nigricans is a strong indicator of insulin resistance.

ACE inhibitor: A blood pressure control drug that prevents the production of angiotensin converting enzyme. This enzyme, if left uncontrolled, prompts the production of angiotensin, a hormone that causes arteries to constrict.

adipocytes: Fat cells.

ARB: Angiotensin receptor blocker, a medication that controls angiotensin by preventing its hormone receptors from working properly. ARBs are another form of blood pressure control drugs.

atherosclerosis: Also known as "hardening of the arteries." It may occur if fatty deposits (plaques) have started lining the artery's interior, the artery walls have calcified, or if high blood pressure has caused artery walls to thicken.

beta blocker: A class of drugs that, by blocking certain substances, relax contractions in the cardiovascular system. Beta blockers are used as angina and blood pressure medications.

blood pressure: The pressure of blood within the arteries created by the pumping of the heart. Blood pressure is highest when the heart beats (systolic pressure), lowest when the heart is at rest (diastolic pressure). Blood pressure is listed as systolic over diastolic, e.g. 120/80.

blood sugar: Glucose in the blood.

BMI: Body mass index, a ratio between height and weight.

carbohydrate: A basic component of food and one of the three major forms of energy sources from which the body draws.

cardiologist: A doctor whose specialty is diseases of the heart.

cholesterol: A waxy substance found in animal fat, essential to the formation of a variety of hormones and vitamins. Cholesterol is carried in the blood as two basic types: LDL, low-density lipoprotein (the "bad" cholesterol), and HDL, high-density lipoprotein (the "good" cholesterol). Cholesterol levels are measured in milligrams per deciliter of blood; ideally, HDL should be over 40 and LDL should be under 70.

cortisol: A hormone that has a major role in the control of glucose and other nutrients. Cortisol levels jump under stress, and high cortisol levels slow metabolism and make you gain weight.

diabetes: diabetes mellitus, "sweet urine": A disease featuring high blood sugar levels and problems in insulin secretion, which reinforce each other. There are two major types of diabetes. The first, type 1, is a congenital condition; the second, type 2 (or adult onset diabetes), is often brought on by obesity and poor diet. Diabetes can lead to atherosclerosis, nerve damage and even death; it's the third leading cause of death in the United States.

diuretic: A substance that prompts the formation of urine.

dyslipidemia: A disorder involving lipid production, particularly an overabundance or deficiency in cholesterol or triglycerides. Metabolic syndrome contributes to dyslipidemia, and dyslipidemia contributes to metabolic syndrome.

endocrinologist: A doctor specializing in hormones and the glands of the endocrine system, which play a paramount role in regulating metabolism, hunger, energy level, sex drive and other bodily functions.

fiber: In a diet, foods or substances difficult to digest. Fiber promotes bowel regularity and appetite satisfaction.

fibrates: A class of cholesterol- and triglyceride-lowering drugs.

free fatty acid: Fatty acids, such as triglycerides, not attached to other molecules. They're a key source of energy for the body, particularly muscle tissue.

glucose: A simple sugar that's carried in the blood, and thus the primary source of energy in the body.

glycemic index: A measure of how fast a food raises glucose in the body. The higher the glycemic index, the faster the glucose is raised. Created in 1981 by Dr. David Jenkins and Dr. Thomas M.S. Wolever.

gout: Disease of elevated uric acid in the blood, characterized by joint pain, kidney stones and fluid retention at the joints.

HDL: High-density lipoprotein, the "good" cholesterol.

hemoglobin A1c: Also known as HbA1c or A1c, a blood protein in red blood cells that has bonded with blood sugar. Since red blood cells can live from 90 to 120 days, hemoglobin A1c stays in the blood for that length of time. A hemoglobin A1c test is useful to determine if a patient has diabetes.

homocysteine: An amino acid, usually produced in the body through eating meat, which serves as a risk factor for cardiovascular disease. High homocysteine levels damage blood vessels, increase risk of clots, and are believed to be linked to Alzheimer's disease.

HOPE trial: A landmark 1990s study that demonstrated the ACE inhibitor ramapril (Altace) could reduce risk of heart attack, stroke, and death from other cardiovascular disease. The trial also indicated that patients who took ramapril had less of a chance of developing type 2 diabetes. HOPE stood for "Heart Outcomes Prevention Evaluation."

hydrogenization: The process of forcing hydrogen atoms into certain foodstuffs, particularly oils, to solidify and even out their consistency. By altering the chemical bonds of these oils, hydrogenization creates trans fats, which in turn cause a variety of health problems.

hyperlipidemia: High fat levels in the blood.

hypertriglyceridemia: High triglyceride levels in the blood.

inflammation: The body's reaction to infection or irritation, such as swelling, redness or pain.

insulin resistance: The declining ability of the body to respond to insulin, the hormone that regulates blood sugar. Insulin resistance arises when rapidly digested carbohydrates and sugars, quickly converted to glucose, cause insulin spikes. As these spikes happen more often, the body gradually requires more glucose to get the same energy, which requires it to produce more insulin. The more insulin released, the less effective it becomes. If left unchecked, a person may succumb to adult onset (type 2) diabetes. Moreover, insulin also promotes the formation of fat – lipogenesis – so the more insulin secreted, the more the body has a tendency to gain weight.

LDL: Low-density lipoprotein, the "bad" cholesterol.

lipid: A fat.

lipogenesis: The formation of fat in the body.

monounsaturated fat: A fat found in olive, canola and peanut oils, so called because of its chemical structure. Monounsaturated fats are liquid at room temperature.

NC: Neck circumference. A large neck circumference may indicate obesity.

niacin: Also known as nicotinic acid or vitamin B_3, a vitamin important to the digestive system, assisting in converting food to energy. It also lowers triglycerides and LDL cholesterol while raising HDL cholesterol.

nutraceutical: A food or food-derived substance that offers health benefits. Nutraceuticals include vitamins, mineral supplements, and herbs and their essential active ingredients.

obesity: In a medical sense, being overweight to a certain degree or higher. Medically, obesity is defined as being 20 percent over your ideal body weight, or having a BMI of more than 30.

omega-3 fatty acid: A type of fatty acid, often found in fish oils and certain high-fiber foods such as flaxseed, that has a number of health benefits — particularly lowering LDL cholesterol. The term "omega-3" comes from the chemical structure of the acid.

pancreatitis: Inflammation of the pancreas, the organ that produces insulin. Related ailments include diabetes and gallstones.

PCOS: Polycystic ovary syndrome, also known as Stein-Leventhal syndrome, a condition with a broad spectrum of symptoms prompted by an excess of the hormone androgen in women. Manifestations include weight gain, insulin resistance, type 2 diabetes, high blood pressure and elevated cholesterol.

plaques: Fatty deposits along artery walls. Plaques can lead to clot formation, stroke, and heart disease.

polyunsaturated fat: A fat primarily found in vegetable oils and fish. Polyunsaturated fats remain liquid at room temperature and are called "polyunsaturated" due to their chemical structures.

saturated fat: A fat, usually animal fat, that is solid or mostly solid at room temperature. Saturated fats are the unhealthy fats, linked to high cholesterol and increased risk of cardiovascular disease.

sleep apnea: An affliction—particularly affecting the overweight—in which a person, while sleeping (and, usually, snoring), stops breathing for a split second because the soft palate constricts the body's airways. The stoppage is usually not enough to fully awaken the sleeper, but it causes body systems to go into overdrive because of the sudden lack of oxygen. The shutdown may happen several times during the night and leaves the sufferer tired and enervated in the morning. Sleep apnea can be treated with a CPAP machine – an instrument that provides a smooth, continuous flow of oxygen to the sleeper – or, in extreme cases, surgery to widen the breathing tube.

sphygmomanometer: A blood pressure gauge.

statin: Also known as HMG-CoA reductase inhibitors, a class of medications that lower cholesterol levels.

thrombogenicity: The likelihood of clots to form in the bloodstream. Medications taken for metabolic syndrome attempt to reduce thrombogenicity.

trans fats: Also known as trans fatty acids, these are the fats formed by liquids, such as vegetable oil, hardened into solids, such as margarine – often by hydrogenating. Trans fats increase LDL, decrease HDL, clog arteries, promote diabetes, and increase the risk of heart disease.

triglycerides: Energy-rich molecules made from fats eaten in foods or created by the body from carbohydrates in food.

urinary microalbumin: A protein found in the urine. Leakage of microalbumin from the kidneys into surrounding tissues may indicate diabetes, high blood pressure, or some immune disorders.

white coat hypertension: When blood pressure is elevated in a doctor's office or other stressful situation. Though once dismissed as nerves, white coat hypertension is now considered a real form of hypertension because it has been found that other stressful situations may also raise blood pressure. Most experts now agree that it should be taken seriously and treated like any other type of hypertension.

WHR: Waist-to-hip ratio, the mathematical relationship between hip circumference and waist circumference. A waist-to-hip ratio of 1.0 or greater is considered to be in the danger zone for obesity.

Index

E

F

M

N

About the Authors

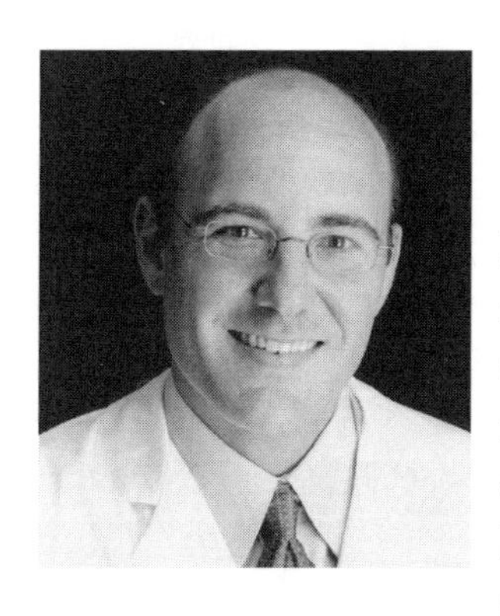

Scott Isaacs, M.D., F.A.C.P., F.A.C.E., is a board-certified endocrinologist in Atlanta, Georgia, where he is Medical Director at Intelligent Health Center, a multidisciplinary center for the treatment of endocrine disorders and obesity. "Endocrinology is the subspecialty of internal medicine dealing with the endocrine glands and hormones and their roles in health and diseases. Because hormones affect virtually every cell and every organ, there are many different symptoms of hormonal imbalance. I always listen to my patients and never discount any symptom, which may be a clue to a hormone problem."

Dr. Isaacs has done research on obesity, stress, and diabetes and has published many articles in peer-reviewed medical journals, including the *Journal of Endocrinology and Metabolism*, *Diabetes Care*, and the *Journal of Critical Care*.

Dr. Isaacs is also a Clinical Instructor of Medicine at Emory University School of Medicine. He attended Emory School of

Medicine and continued on at Emory for his residency and fellowship in endocrinology, diabetes, and metabolism. He gives many lectures on the subject of hormones and obesity, speaking to groups in the community as well as at major events and conferences throughout the United States. He also trains other doctors in the field.

Dr. Isaacs has been quoted in many national publications, including *Better Homes and Gardens, Better Health and Living, Women's Health and Fitness, Prevention, The Atlanta Journal-Constitution, The Chicago Tribune, Men's Health, Fitness Magazine, Glamour, Women's World, First Health, Florida International Magazine*, and many others. He has given expert commentary on several radio and television news programs including local NBC, ABC, CBS, and Fox News affiliates, *CNN Headline News*, and has appeared as a weight loss expert on TBS Superstation's *Movie and a Makeover*.

Dr. Isaacs is also the author of *Hormonal Balance: Understanding Hormones, Weight and Your Metabolism* (Bull Publishing, 2002) and *A Simple Guide to Thyroid Disorders: From Diagnosis to Treatment* (Addicus Books, 2003). Dr. Isaacs is an officer of the Georgia chapter of the American Association of Clinical Endocrinologists and is the medical advisor for Cushing's Understanding, Support, and Help Organization. Dr. Isaacs is a Diplomat of the American Board of Bariatric Medicine, a Fellow of the American College of Physicians (FACP), and a Fellow of the American College of Endocrinology (FACE).

Dr. Isaacs may be reached through his Web site: **www.intelligenthealthcenter.com**.

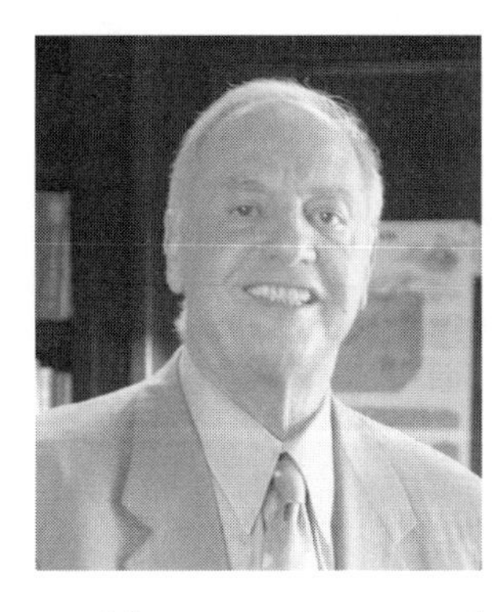

Frederic J. Vagnini, M.D., a cardiovascular surgeon, is medical director of the Heart, Diabetes, and Weight Loss Centers of New York City.

After graduation from St. Louis University School of Medicine in 1963, Dr. Vagnini underwent eight years of postdoctorate internship and residency during which he studied vascular, heart, and lung surgery at the Downstate Medical Center, Brooklyn, New York, and Columbia Presbyterian Medical Center, New York City. After he completed his training, Dr. Vagnini served in the United States Army as a lieutenant colonel and subsequently entered into private practice on Long Island, New York. For the next twenty-five years, Dr. Vagnini practiced as a heart, lung, and blood vessel surgeon. He has performed surgery on thousands of patients with heart and blood vessel disease.

As his career continued, Dr. Vagnini became interested in health education, preventive medicine, and clinical nutrition. Because of his experience in the area of heart disease and nutrition, he became a frequent guest speaker and has appeared numerous times on local and national radio and television. Dr. Vagnini presently hosts a live call-in show on WOR Radio 710 AM: *The Heart Show.* Dr. Vagnini formerly hosted a national health program on Fox Television.

Dr. Vagnini is the coauthor of the *New York Times* bestseller, *The Carbohydrate Addict's Healthy Heart Program* (Ballantine Books, 1999). He is author of *The Side Effects Bible* (Broadway Books, 2005) and *30 Minutes a Day to a Healthy Heart* (Reader's

Digest Books, 2005). He has written numerous articles for both consumer and scientific publications. He also publishes a monthly newsletter, *Cardiovascular Wellness Newsletter*, that covers current health news issues with commentary.

Dr. Vagnini is certified by the American Board of Surgery and the American Board of Thoracic Surgery. He is an active member of numerous medical societies and associations. Dr. Vagnini can be reached through his Web site: **www.vagnini.com.**

Other Consumer Health Titles from Addicus Books

Visit our online catalog at www.AddicusBooks.com

After Mastectomy—Healing Physically and Emotionally	$14.95
Cancers of the Mouth and Throat—A Patient's Guide to Treatment	$14.95
Cataracts: A Patient's Guide to Treatment	$14.95
Colon & Rectal Cancer—A Patient's Guide to Treatment	$14.95
Coping with Psoriasis—A Patient's Guide to Treatment	$14.95
Coronary Heart Disease—A Guide to Diagnosis and Treatment	$15.95
Exercising Through Your Pregnancy	$17.95
The Fertility Handbook—A Guide to Getting Pregnant	$14.95
The Healing Touch—Keeping the Doctor/Patient Relationship Alive Under Managed Care	$9.95
The Macular Degeneration Source Book	$14.95
LASIK—A Guide to Laser Vision Correction	$14.95
Living with P.C.O.S.—Polycystic Ovarian Syndrome	$14.95
Lung Cancer—A Guide to Treatment & Diagnosis	$14.95
The Macular Degeneration Source Book	$14.95
The Non-Surgical Facelift Book—A Guide to Facial Rejuvenation Procedures	$19.95
Overcoming Postpartum Depression and Anxiety	$14.95
A Patient's Guide to Dental Implants	$14.95
Prescription Drug Addiction—The Hidden Epidemic	$15.95
Prostate Cancer—A Patient's Guide to Treatment	$14.95
Simple Changes: The Boomer's Guide to a Healthier, Happier Life	$9.95
A Simple Guide to Thyroid Disorders	$14.95
Straight Talk About Breast Cancer—From Diagnosis to Recovery	$14.95
The Stroke Recovery Book—A Guide for Patients and Families	$14.95
The Surgery Handbook—A Guide to Understanding Your Operation	$14.95
Understanding Lumpectomy—A Treatment Guide for Breast Cancer	$14.95
Understanding Parkinson's Disease—A Self-Help Guide	$14.95

Organizations, associations, corporations, hospitals, and other groups may qualify for special discounts when ordering more than 24 copies. For more information, please contact the Special Sales Department at Addicus Books. Phone (402) 330-7493. Email: Addicusbks@aol.com.

Please send:

________ copies of ____

(Title of book)

at $ ____________ each TOTAL: ________________

Nebraska residents add 5% sales tax ________________

Shipping/Handling

$4.00 postage for first book.

$1.10 postage for each additional book ________________

TOTAL ENCLOSED: ________________

Name ____

Address ____

City ____________________________ State __________ Zip ____________

☐ **Visa** ☐ **MasterCard** ☐ **American Express**

Credit card number __________________ Expiration date ________________

Order by credit card, personal check or money order. Send to: